Melanoma

Susana Ortiz-Urda · Wilson Ho · Albert Lee

Melanoma

From Diagnosis to Therapy

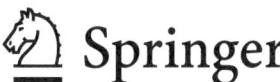

Susana Ortiz-Urda
Department of Dermatology
University of California, San Francisco
San Francisco, CA, USA

Wilson Ho
Department of Dermatology
University of California, San Francisco
San Francisco, CA, USA

Albert Lee
Department of Dermatology
University of California, San Francisco
San Francisco, CA, USA

ISBN 978-3-031-59127-3   ISBN 978-3-031-59128-0   (eBook)
https://doi.org/10.1007/978-3-031-59128-0

© The Editor(s) (if applicable) and The Author(s), under exclusive license to Springer Nature Switzerland AG 2024

This work is subject to copyright. All rights are solely and exclusively licensed by the Publisher, whether the whole or part of the material is concerned, specifically the rights of translation, reprinting, reuse of illustrations, recitation, broadcasting, reproduction on microfilms or in any other physical way, and transmission or information storage and retrieval, electronic adaptation, computer software, or by similar or dissimilar methodology now known or hereafter developed.

The use of general descriptive names, registered names, trademarks, service marks, etc. in this publication does not imply, even in the absence of a specific statement, that such names are exempt from the relevant protective laws and regulations and therefore free for general use.

The publisher, the authors and the editors are safe to assume that the advice and information in this book are believed to be true and accurate at the date of publication. Neither the publisher nor the authors or the editors give a warranty, expressed or implied, with respect to the material contained herein or for any errors or omissions that may have been made. The publisher remains neutral with regard to jurisdictional claims in published maps and institutional affiliations.

This Springer imprint is published by the registered company Springer Nature Switzerland AG
The registered company address is: Gewerbestrasse 11, 6330 Cham, Switzerland

If disposing of this product, please recycle the paper.

Preface

The purpose of this book is to provide training for residents and physicians while also educating interested patients and family members on the crucial concepts related to the diagnosis and treatment of melanoma. It is also to serve as a concise yet comprehensive guide for patients seeking knowledge on important topics within the broad range of melanoma research and its clinical applications.

My residents inspired me to write this book. The idea for this project started with my lectures and the realization that there is much more that I wanted to cover. It has been expanded to include everything including melanoma diagnosis, treatment, types of melanomas, and the nuances in clinical practice.

I would like to dedicate this book to my mother and all the heroes who have endured this disease.

Susana Ortiz-Urda, MD, PhD, MBA
Wilson Ho
Albert Lee

Contents

1 Melanoma Staging 1
    Melanoma Staging Process 1
    Tumor Characteristics (T) 1
        Possible T Values 2
    Lymph Nodes (N) 2
        Possible *N* Values 3
    Metastatic Spread (M) 3
        Possible M Values 3
    Stage Grouping 4
    Stage and Tumor Characteristics (TNM) 4
        Stage Group 0 4
        Stage Group I 4
        Stage Group II 4
        Stage Group III 5
        Stage Group IV 6
    References 6

2 Molecular Diagnosis of Melanoma 7
    Mutations in the Pathogenesis of Melanoma 7
    Mutation Testing 10
    Effects of Mutations on Therapy 10
    Clinical Application of CGH/FISH for Melanoma 12
    References 13

3 Familial Melanoma 17
    Genetic Mutations 17
    Genetic Testing and Counseling 18
    References 19

4 Treatment for Stages I–III 23
    Stage 0 Treatment 23
        Wide Local Excision [1–7] 23
    Stage IA Treatment 23
        Wide Local Excision 23

		Stage IB–II Treatment.	23
		Wide Local Excision and Sentinel Lymph Node (SLN) Biopsy	23
		Stage III Treatment	25
		Baseline Imaging, Primary Treatment, and Adjuvant Treatment and/or Observation	25
		References.	26
5	**Treatment for Regionally Advanced and In-transit Melanoma**		29
	In-transit Melanoma		29
	Therapy Options		29
	Isolated Limb Perfusion (ILP)		30
	Isolated Limb Infusion (ILI)		31
	Intralesional Therapy		32
	References.		33
6	**Treatment for Stage IV**		37
	Introduction		37
	Surgery		37
	Brain Metastases		38
	Targeted Therapy		38
	Immunotherapy		39
	Combination Immunotherapy		40
	Combination Targeted and Immunotherapy		41
	Choosing Therapy		42
	References.		42
7	**Side Effects of Melanoma Therapy**		47
	Targeted Therapy		47
	Immune Checkpoint Inhibitors		48
	References.		49
8	**Pediatric Melanoma**		51
	Clinical Presentation		51
	Risk Factors		53
	Prognosis		53
	Management		54
	References.		54
9	**Melanoma and Pregnancy**		57
	Introduction		57
	Melanoma During Pregnancy		57
	Treatment for Patients with Advanced PAM		58
	Melanoma During the Postpartum Period		59
	Melanoma Diagnosed Prior to Pregnancy		59
	Influence of Hormones on Melanoma		59
	References.		59

10 Mucosal Melanoma ... 63
Head and Neck ... 64
Genitourinary ... 64
Anorectal ... 65
Molecular Biology of Mucosal Melanoma ... 65
Management of Primary Disease ... 66
Adjuvant Therapy ... 66
Systemic Therapy ... 67
References ... 68

11 Uveal Melanoma ... 71
Clinical High-Risk Features ... 72
    Older Age ... 72
    Largest Tumor Diameter ... 72
    Ciliary Body Involvement ... 72
    Extraocular Extension ... 73
    Diffuse Pattern ... 73
    Ring Melanoma ... 73
    Optic Nerve Involvement ... 74
Histological High-Risk Features ... 74
    Cell Type ... 74
    Mean Diameter of the Ten Largest Nucleoli ... 74
    High Mitotic Rate ... 75
    Microcirculation ... 75
    Pigmentation ... 76
    Inflammation ... 76
Immunohistochemical Markers ... 76
Molecular Pathology ... 77
Molecular Pathway Defects in Primary UM ... 78
Chromosomal Alterations in Primary UM ... 78
Molecular Techniques Used for Prognostication in Primary UM ... 79
Molecular Alterations in UM Metastases ... 79
Scope of Prognostication ... 80
Treatment Modalities ... 80
References ... 81

12 Conjunctival Melanoma ... 87
Terminology and Classification of Early Lesions ... 87
Conjunctival Melanoma (CoM) ... 88
Genetic Abnormalities ... 89
Staging ... 90
Management ... 91
Prognosis ... 93
References ... 94

13 Minority Melanoma Paradox ... 99
Melanoma Development in Non-White Populations ... 100
Clinical Presentation ... 101
Prevention ... 103
Conclusion ... 104
References ... 105

14 Melanoma Risk with Immunomodulators ... 109
Introduction ... 109
Melanoma Development in Immunosuppressed Patients ... 109
Increased Melanoma Risk ... 110
No Increased Melanoma Risk ... 111
Inconclusive Melanoma Risk ... 111
Risk of Melanoma Progression or Recurrence ... 112
Melanoma Prognosis during Immunosuppressant Treatment ... 112
Conclusion ... 113
References ... 113

15 Dermoscopy ... 117
Dermoscopy Background ... 117
Features of Melanocytic Lesions ... 119
Nonmelanocytic Lesions ... 120
    Ink Spot Lentigo ... 120
    Solar Lentigo ... 120
    Seborrheic Keratosis ... 121
    Basal Cell Carcinoma ... 121
    Sebaceous Gland Hyperplasia ... 122
    Dermatofibroma ... 122
    Vascular Lesions ... 123
    Squamous Cell Carcinoma ... 123
Stratifying Risk of Melanocytic Lesions ... 124
Benign Melanocytic Lesions ... 125
    Congenital Nevus ... 125
    Acquired Nevus ... 125
    Blue Nevus ... 126
    Combined Nevus ... 126
    Unna and Miescher Nevi ... 126
Higher-Risk Melanocytic Lesions ... 127
    Recurrent Nevus ... 127
    Dysplastic Nevus ... 128
    Nevus Spilus ... 129
    Spitz Nevus ... 130
Melanoma ... 130
    Melanoma In Situ ... 130
    Lentigo Maligna and Lentigo Maligna Melanoma ... 130
    Superficial Spreading and Nodular Melanoma ... 131

	Hypomelanotic and Amelanotic Melanoma	133
	Cutaneous Metastatic Melanoma	134
	Acral Melanoma	134
	Subungual Melanoma	135
	Mucosal Melanoma	136
	Conclusion	136
	References	136
16	**Risk Factors for Melanoma Development**	143
	Risk Factors	143
	Role of Dermoscopy	144
	Role of Total Body Photography (TBP)	144
	Occupational Risk Factors	145
	References	145
Index		147

Melanoma Staging

Melanoma is the most aggressive and deadly form of skin cancer and develops melanocytes as opposed to other epithelial cells. Although it accounts for only 1% of skin cancers, it causes the majority of skin cancer-related deaths [1].

Melanoma Staging Process

Melanoma tumors are staged with the *TNM staging method*. TNM stands for **T**umor characteristics: thickness and ulceration of the tumor, **N**odal presence: whether the melanoma has spread to nearby lymph nodes, and **M**etastasis: whether the melanoma tumor has spread to any other organs. The current version is outlined in the *AJCC 8th Edition Cancer Staging Manual* [2] and includes an updated classification framework. It was implemented in the United States on January 1, 2018.

Below is a more detailed explanation of the TNM staging process [2–7]:

Tumor Characteristics (T)

T is based on tumor thickness and ulceration status. Before the 8th edition, mitotic rate was also included and is still an important prognostic factor. They are explained below:

1. **Thickness (Breslow depth)**. How deeply the tumor has penetrated the skin. Thickness is measured in millimeters (mm) to the nearest 0.1 mm. For example:
    (a) 1 mm = 0.04 in., or less than 1/16 in. (about equal to the edge of a penny)
    (b) 2 mm = between 1/16 and 1/8 in. (about equal to the edge of a nickel)
    (c) 4 mm = between 1/8 and 1/4 in. (about equal to the edges of two nickels)
2. **Ulceration**. When the epidermis (or top layer of skin) that covers a portion of the primary melanoma is not intact. Ulceration can only be seen under a microscope, not by the naked eye.

© The Author(s), under exclusive license to Springer Nature Switzerland AG 2024
S. Ortiz-Urda et al., *Melanoma*, https://doi.org/10.1007/978-3-031-59128-0_1

3. **Mitotic count (rate)** is a secondary characteristic that describes how quickly the tumor cells are dividing. Mitotic count is calculated by a pathologist, who counts the average number of actively dividing cells present in the biopsy sample. Though not used to determine T stage in the 8th edition, it is still an important prognostic factor and should be evaluated.

Possible T Values

- **TX**: The thickness of the primary tumor cannot be assessed.
- **Tis**: Melanoma in situ. (The tumor remains in the epidermis, the outermost layer of skin.)
- **T0**: No evidence of the primary tumor.
- **T1a**: The melanoma is less than 0.8 mm thick without ulceration.
- **T1b**: The melanoma is between 0.8 and 1.0 mm or less than 0.8 mm thick with ulceration.
- **T2a**: The melanoma is between >1.0 and 2.0 mm thick without ulceration.
- **T2b**: The melanoma is between >1.0 and 2.0 mm thick with ulceration.
- **T3a**: The melanoma is between >2.0 and 4.0 mm thick without ulceration.
- **T3b**: The melanoma is between >2.0 and 4.0 mm thick with ulceration.
- **T4a**: The melanoma is thicker than 4.0 mm without ulceration.
- **T4b**: The melanoma is thicker than 4.0 mm with ulceration.

Lymph Nodes (N)

N is based on whether the tumor has moved to the lymph nodes and the degree of movement. Sentinel lymph node biopsy must be done to analyze nodal movement, but it is not always performed.

Some Relevant Terms Used in Nodal Staging Include
1. **Clinically occult**. Unable to be clinically detected (previously termed microscopic in 7th edition)
2. **Clinically detected**. Visible on imaging tests or able to be physically (previously termed macroscopic in 7th edition)
3. **In-transit metastases**. Clinically evident metastases that are greater than 2 cm from the primary melanoma but have not reached the first draining lymph node
4. **Satellite metastases**. Visible metastases occurring within 2 cm of the primary melanoma
5. **Microsatellite metastases**. Discontinuous microscopic metastases adjacent to primary melanoma
6. **Matted nodes**. Lymph nodes that are clumped or adhered together

Possible N Values

Clinical Staging (Without Sentinel Lymph Node Biopsy)
- **NX**: Nearby (regional) lymph nodes cannot be assessed.
- **N0**: No spread to nearby lymph nodes.
- **N1**: Spread to one nearby lymph node, OR presence of in-transit, satellite, and/or microsatellite metastases without nodal involvement.
- **N2**: Spread to two or three nearby lymph nodes, OR presence of in-transit, satellite, and/or microsatellite metastases involving one lymph node.
- **N3**: Spread to four or more lymph nodes, OR presence of in-transit, satellite, and/or microsatellite metastases involving two or more lymph nodes OR presence of matted nodes.

Following a lymph node biopsy, the *pathological stage* can be determined using the additional information:

- **Any Na (N1a, N2a, or N3a)**: The melanoma is in the lymph node(s) but is clinically occult.
- **Any Nb (N1b, N2b, or N3b)**: The melanoma is in the lymph node(s) and at least one node large enough to clinically detected. Matted nodes also fall under this category.
- **Any Nc (N1c, N2c, N3c)**: The melanoma has spread to nearby skin (satellite/microsatellite metastases) or has spread to skin lymphatic channels around the tumor (in-transit metastases).

Metastatic Spread (M)

M is based on whether the melanoma tumor has spread or metastasized to other organs.

Possible M Values

- **M0**: No distant metastasis
- **M1a**: Metastasis to skin, soft tissue including muscle, or lymph nodes in distant parts of the body
- **M1b**: Metastasis to the lungs
- **M1c**: Metastasis to other organs not part of the central nervous system
- **M1d**: Metastasis to the central nervous system

An additional suffix is assigned based on LDH levels: (0) if LDH is not elevated, (1) if LDH is elevated, and blank if LDH levels are unknown. For example, a melanoma grouped as M1a with non-elevated LDH levels would be noted as M1a(0).

Stage Grouping

Once the T, N, and M groups have been determined, they are combined to give an overall stage, using Roman numerals I to IV (1–4), which may be further subdivided. This process is called *stage grouping*. In general, patients with lower staging have a better outlook for recovery or long-term survival. The overall stage grouping value is based on pathological TNM staging.

The final stage grouping can be efficiently narrowed by using the following to determine the appropriate starting point:

1. If a patient is M1, having metastatic spread → *Stage Group IV*
2. If a patient is N1 or greater, having nodal involvement → *Stage Group III*
3. If a patient is T2b or greater, meeting thickness and ulceration criteria → *Stage Group II*
4. Otherwise, begin at *Stage Group I* for T1a to T2a and *Stage Group 0* for Tis.

Stage and Tumor Characteristics (TNM)

Stage Group 0

Stage 0: Tis, N0, M0: The melanoma is in situ, meaning that it is in the epidermis but has not spread to the dermis (lower layer).

Stage Group I

Stage IA: T1a or pT1b, N0, M0: The melanoma is less than or equal to 1.0 mm in thickness. It has not been found in lymph nodes or distant organs.

Stage IB: cT1b or T2a, N0, M0: The melanoma is less than or equal to 1.0 mm in thickness with ulceration OR is between >1.0 and 2.0 mm in thickness without ulceration. It has not been found in lymph nodes or distant organs.

Stage Group II

Stage IIA: T2b or T3a, N0, M0: The melanoma is between >1.0 and 2.0 mm in thickness with ulceration OR is between >2.0 and 4.0 mm without ulceration. It has not been found in lymph nodes or distant organs.

Stage IIB: T3b or T4a, N0, M0: The melanoma is between >2.0 and 4.0 mm with ulceration OR is thicker than 4.0 mm without ulceration. It has not been found in lymph nodes or distant organs.

Stage IIC: T4b, N0, M0: The melanoma is thicker than 4.0 mm with ulceration. It has not been found in lymph nodes or distant organs.

Stage and Tumor Characteristics (TNM)

Stage Group III

Stage IIIA: T1a/b to T2a, N1a or N2a, M0: The melanoma is less than or equal to 2mm thick without ulceration or less than 0.8 mm thick with ulceration. It has spread to one to three lymph nodes near the affected skin area, but the nodes are not enlarged, and the melanoma is clinically occult. There is no distant spread.

Stage IIIB: One of the Following Applies
- **T0, N1b/c, M0**: No primary tumor is evident. The melanoma has spread to one nearby lymph node near the affected skin area and is clinically detectable OR has spread to nearby skin or lymphatic channels around the original tumor, but not to the lymph nodes. There is no distant spread.
- **T1a/b to T2a, N1b/c or N2b, M0**: The melanoma is less than 1.0 mm with or without ulceration or between 1.0 and 2.0 mm without ulceration. It has spread to one to three lymph nodes near the affected skin area and is clinically detectable OR has spread to nearby skin or lymphatic channels around the original tumor, but not to the lymph nodes. There is no distant spread.
- **T2b or T3a, N1a to N2b, M0**: The melanoma is between 1.0 and 2.0 mm with ulceration or 2.0–4.0 mm without ulceration. It has spread to one to three lymph nodes near the affected skin area and may be clinically occult OR has spread to nearby skin or lymphatic channels around the original tumor, but not to the lymph nodes. There is no distant spread.

Stage IIIC: One of the Following Applies
- **T0, N2b/c or N3b/c, M0**: No primary tumor is evident. Disease has spread to two or more nearby lymph nodes near the affected skin area, is clinically detectable, and may have spread to very small areas of nearby skin or has spread to lymphatic channels around the tumor. There is no distant spread.
- **T1a to T3a, N2c or N3a/b/c, M0**: The melanoma is less than 2.0 mm with or without ulceration or between 2.0 and 4.0 mm without ulceration. It has spread to four or more lymph nodes OR has spread to nearby skin or lymphatic channels around the tumor and to nearby lymph node(s). There is no distant spread.
- **T3b or T4a, any N > N0, M0**: The melanoma is between 2.0 and 4.0 mm with ulceration or greater than 4.0 mm without ulceration. It has spread to at least one lymph node OR to nearby skin or lymphatic channels around the original tumor. There is no distant spread.
- **T4b, N1a to N2c, M0**: The melanoma is thicker than 4.0 mm with ulceration. It has spread to one to three nearby lymph nodes, OR to nearby lymph nodes that are clumped together, OR has spread to nearby skin or lymphatic channels around the original tumor and to at most one nearby lymph node. There is no distant spread.

Stage IIID: T4b, N3a/b/c, M0: The melanoma is thicker than 4.0 mm with ulceration. It has spread to four or more lymph nodes OR has spread to nearby skin or lymphatic channels around the original tumor and to at least two lymph nodes. There is no distant spread.

Stage Group IV

Stage IV: Any T, any N, M1(a, b, c, or d): The melanoma has spread beyond the original area of skin and nearby lymph nodes to other organs such as the lung, liver, or brain or to distant areas of the skin, subcutaneous tissue, or distant lymph nodes. Neither spread to nearby lymph nodes nor thickness is considered in this stage, but typically the melanoma is thick and has also spread to the lymph node.

References

1. American Cancer Society. Cancer facts & figures 2019. Atlanta: American Cancer Society; 2019. https://www.cancer.org/research/cancer-facts-statistics/all-cancer-facts-figures/cancer-facts-figures-2019.html. Accessed 27 July 2020.
2. Amin MB, Edge SB, Greene FL, et al. AJCC cancer staging manual. 8th ed. New York: Springer; 2017. p. 563–85.
3. Balch CM, Buzaid AC, Soong S-J, Atkins MB, Cascinelli N, Coit DG, et al. Final version of the American Joint Committee on Cancer Staging System for cutaneous melanoma. J Clin Oncol. 2001;19(16):3635–48.
4. Balch CM, Gershenwald JE, Soong S, Thompson JF, Atkins MB, Byrd DR, et al. Final version of 2009 AJCC Melanoma Staging and Classification. J Clin Oncol. 2009;27(36):6199–206.
5. Balch CM, Soong S-J, Gershenwald JE, Thompson JF, Reintgen DS, Cascinelli N, et al. Prognostic factors analysis of 17,600 melanoma patients: validation of the American Joint Committee on cancer melanoma staging system. J Clin Oncol. 2001;19(16):3622–34.
6. Balch CM, Buzaid AC, Atkins MB, Cascinelli N, Coit DG, Fleming ID, et al. A new American Joint Committee on Cancer staging system for cutaneous melanoma. Cancer. 2000;88(6):1484–91.
7. Gershenwald JE, Scolyer RA, Hess KR, Sondak VK, Long GV, Ross MI, et al. Melanoma staging: evidence-based changes in the American Joint Committee on Cancer eighth edition cancer staging manual. CA Cancer J Clin. 2017;67(6):472–92.

Molecular Diagnosis of Melanoma

There is a clear role of UV radiation in melanoma development, as invasive melanoma has more UV-induced mutations than in nevi [1, 2]. It is one of the factors leading to a number of genetic and genomic mutations identified to be drivers of melanoma pathogenesis. A majority are point mutations, but there are also larger genomic aberrations. Whole-genome sequencing analysis shows that certain genes are most susceptible to mutation in cutaneous melanoma including BRAF, cyclin-dependent kinase N2A (CDKN2A), NRAS, and TP53 [3].

Mutations in the Pathogenesis of Melanoma

BRAF is a proto-oncogenic kinase involved in cell proliferation via the mitogen-activated protein kinase (MAPK) pathway signaling after activation by a RAS family protein. Moreover, 50–60% of cutaneous melanomas carry a mutation in BRAF, with the most common (79%) being a valine-to-glutamate substitution at codon 600 (BRAF V600E) [4, 5]. Less common mutations in BRAF include substitutions of valine to lysine (12%), to arginine (5%), or to methionine (4%) [5, 6]. BRAF mutant melanomas are associated with a superficial spreading or nodular type, truncal location, and patients less than 50 years old [7].

The second protein most frequently mutated in melanoma (15–30% of melanomas) is NRAS, specifically in codon 12, 13, or 61, and these mutations are largely mutually exclusive from BRAF mutations [8]. The most common is at codon 61, specifically Q61L, and other less common mutations include Q61R and Q61H [9]. NRAS mutation is associated with thicker tumors, higher rates of mitosis, and worse clinical outcome compared to tumors with BRAF mutation and tumors with wild-type BRAF/NRAS [10]. The effect of BRAF or NRAS mutation is increased or constitutive MAPK activation with subsequent growth and proliferation, independent of upstream signaling. Although these mutations can lead to aberrant growth, additional mutations are required for malignant transformation [11]. This can explain the fact that up to 80% of benign nevi can harbor BRAF mutations but are limited by oncogene-mediated activation of cell senescence [12, 13]. Likewise, up to 81% of congenital melanocytic nevi harbor a mutation in NRAS [14].

Mutations in tumor suppressors such as PTEN, CDKN2A, TP53, or TERT are required to allow the uncontrolled cellular proliferation seen in melanoma [15–17]. PTEN mutations are detected in 10–30% of cutaneous melanomas and are associated with the vertical growth phase melanoma and with metastases [18, 19]. The tumor suppressors p16INK4a and p14-ARF are two proteins that are encoded by the CDKN2A gene locus, which is mutated in 15% of familial melanomas, and somatic defects in the gene can be found in up to 90% of melanomas [15]. Of genetic abnormalities identified in families with multiple cases of melanoma, CDKN2A was the most common, followed by CDK4 [20–22].

Mutations in the tumor suppressor PTEN are more often found in conjunction with BRAF mutations compared to cell lines with NRAS mutations [23]. PTEN works by inhibiting the PI3K/AKT pathway, a pathway that is important in several cancers including melanoma, breast cancer, and prostate cancer.

Neurofibromin 1 (NF1) mutations appear to a role in some melanomas, as 15–18% of melanomas have nearly absent neurofibromin expression [24]. The wild-type NF1 protein converts active RAS-GTP to inactive RAS-GDP to inhibit MAPK signaling [25]. Therefore, a loss-of-function mutation in NF1 leads to increased activation of the MAPK and PI3K pathways [24, 25]. Melanomas can be divided into subtypes by mutations leading to either loss of NF1 activity, increased BRAF activity, or increased NRAS activity and a group of melanomas that are wild type for all three (Fig. 2.1).

The receptor tyrosine kinase, KIT, is involved in melanoma proliferation and survival through activation of the MAPK and PI3K pathways. Somatic mutations

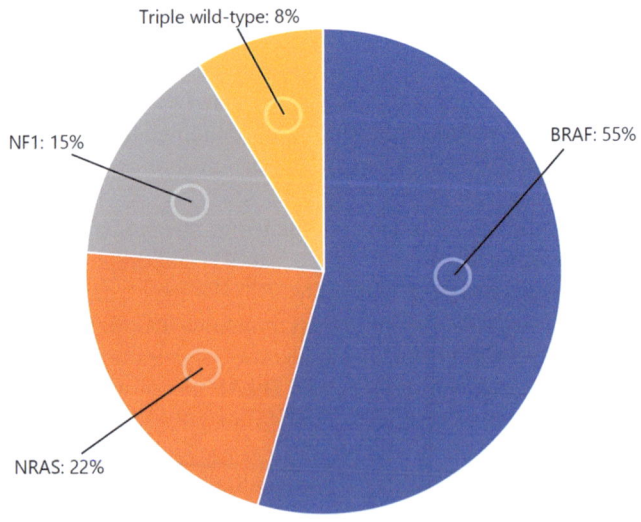

Percentages calculated from The Cancer Genome Atlas (TCGA) mutation data on 469 cutaneous melanomas

Fig. 2.1 Frequencies of the common driver mutations in melanoma

leading to increased activation are found in 2–8% of malignant melanomas and occur more frequently in acral melanomas, mucosal melanomas, and melanomas arising on intermittently sun-exposed skin [26–28].

Mutations in the promoter region of telomerase reverse transcriptase (TERT) have been observed in 71% of melanomas and represent a two to four fold increase activity [29]. TERT is a catalytic subunit of telomerase, whose function is to prevent shortening of telomeres and subsequent cellular senescence. The TERT mutation is more often found in metastatic tumors at 85% compared to primary melanomas at 33% [30]. The specific mutation present may affect outcome with a c.−146C > T mutation having significantly worse progression-free survival than a c.−124C > T mutation (median 5.4 vs 9.5 months, respectively) [31].

TP53 mutations are relative uncommon in melanoma tumors at 19% compared to other cancers, suggesting that melanomas develop ways to overcome its tumor suppressive effects [18, 32]. Rather than acting directly on TP53, mutations in the other elements of the p53 pathway are more common, such as in the p53 negative regulators MDM2 and MDM4 [33, 34]; the homolog p63, which is in the p53 family [35]; and the p53 inhibitor iASPP [32, 36].

Mutations in the genes GNAQ and GNA11, coding for the alpha subunit of G proteins, are found commonly in uveal melanoma, infrequently in blue nevi, and rarely in cutaneous melanoma [37]. This subunit serves as an important switch for signaling, as bound GTP leads to an active state, while hydrolysis to GDP leads to an inactive state. Mutations that block the hydrolysis of GTP to GDP lead to aberrant activation of downstream pathways including the MAPK pathway (Fig. 2.2).

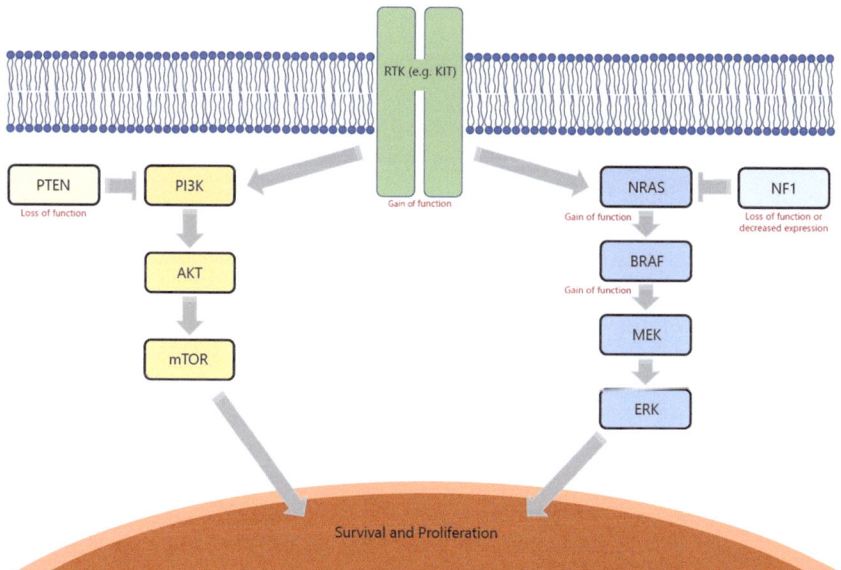

Fig. 2.2 Simplified overview of the MAPK and PI3K pathways and the common types of mutations in melanoma

Mutation Testing

Currently, tumors are only routinely evaluated for the presence of a BRAF V600 mutation in the clinical setting because it can determine whether one of the first-line treatment strategies can be used [16]. Tests for the presence of BRAF mutations fall into categories of companion diagnostic devices or laboratory-developed tests. Companion diagnostic devices are tested and reviewed by the FDA and US Centers for Medicare and Medicaid Services and are often codeveloped with a corresponding therapeutic product for safe and effective use [38]. Current FDA-approved companion diagnostic devices for BRAF mutations in melanoma and their corresponding therapies include FoundationOne CDx (dabrafenib, vemurafenib, or combinations with trametinib), THXID BRAF Kit (encorafenib with binimetinib or dabrafenib with trametinib), and cobas® 4800 BRAF V600 Mutation Test (vemurafenib with or without cobimetinib) [39]. The cobas® 4800 BRAF V600 Mutation Test and THXID BRAF Kit are based on real-time PCR, while the FoundationOne CDx is a next-generation sequencing test and can detect mutations in an additional 324 genes [39].

Laboratory developed tests are typically designed by a hospital or research laboratory. They may be used if they are reviewed by the US Centers for Medicare and Medicaid Services and used in a Clinical Laboratory Improvement Amendments (CLIA)-certified laboratory [38]. The FDA seems to also be increasing regulation of laboratory tests as well because of increasing test complexity [40, 41]. Laboratory tests use various sequencing techniques and immunohistochemistry assays with VE1 antibodies specific for the BRAF V600E mutation [36]. One example is the UCSF500 test, which analyzes nearly 500 genes including most known genes and is periodically updated.

Effects of Mutations on Therapy

Systemic therapy options for melanoma are based on immunotherapy or kinase inhibitors, with kinase inhibitors providing a higher response rate, but immunotherapy providing more long-term durable responses [42–44]. Vemurafenib and dabrafenib are two BRAF inhibitor (targeted therapy) drugs used to treat advanced-stage melanoma with a known BRAF V600E mutation and BRAF V600E/K mutations, respectively [38]. Critically, BRAF mutation status testing is necessary before starting therapy with a BRAF inhibitor because it may lead to paradoxical activation of MAPK signaling in BRAF wild-type tumors [45].

Compared to BRAF inhibitor monotherapy, combination with a MEK inhibitor has led to high response rates (70%) and rapid control of symptoms, with a progression-free survival of approximately 12 months [46–48]. The combination therapy of dabrafenib and trametinib appears to have reduced adverse events compared to the combination of vemurafenib and cobimetinib [49]. The targets of these therapies are shown in Fig. 2.3. Therapies will be discussed further in Chap. 6.

While not currently routinely tested, evaluation of tumor genomic alterations in NRAS, NF1, KIT, CDKN2A, or PTEN can benefit patients for experimental

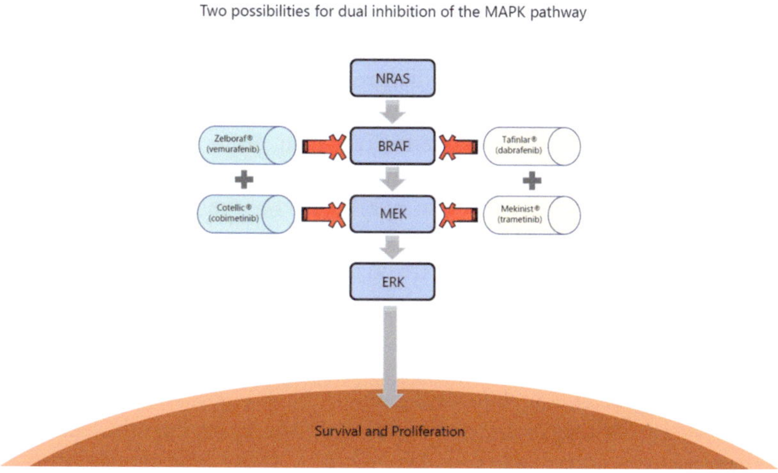

Fig. 2.3 MAPK phosphorylation cascade with inhibition sites of the combination of BRAF and MEK inhibitors

approaches or clinical trials [16]. Determining the mutation status may also be helpful for stratifying risk in challenging melanocytic lesions, such as atypical Spitz tumors [50].

In some situations, testing for a mutation in KIT in melanoma aids in determining whether using a KIT inhibitor may be helpful. The KIT inhibitor, imatinib, is regarded as a second-line treatment for melanoma, after immune checkpoint therapy and BRAF-targeted therapy, because of a response rate of less than 50% in patients with KIT alterations [51–54]. An activating KIT mutation such as L576P or K642E has been shown to be more predictive of a better response to imatinib than copy number gains [55, 56]. There does seem to be some promise and future randomized control trials may help determine its preferred place in therapy options. In particular, the combination of imatinib with immunotherapy may improve response rates with tolerable adverse effects [36, 37].

Testing for PTEN may help predict response to therapies. Specifically, a preclinical study has shown that PTEN loss is associated with decreased infiltration by $CD8^+$ T cells [57]. Additional studies may demonstrate whether this plays a role in the variability seen in the response rates to immune checkpoint inhibitors. Patients treated with dabrafenib for melanoma harboring a PTEN mutation also showed lower progression-free survival of 18.3 weeks compared to 32.1 weeks in patients who had nonmutant PTEN [58]. This may be due to the role of PTEN as an endogenous inhibitor of the PI3K/AKT pathway, which can be activated when some melanomas develop resistance to BRAF inhibitor therapy. As genetic testing becomes increasingly available and therapies increasingly personalized, finding the associations between mutations present and patient outcomes will continue to be key in improving therapies.

Clinical Application of CGH/FISH for Melanoma

Consultant pathologists may strongly disagree on the malignancy of a melanocytic lesion in 20–30% of cases, so testing for chromosomal aberrations as an ancillary technique can be useful for differentiating nevi from melanomas [59, 60]. Fluorescence in situ hybridization (FISH) uses labeled probes targeting specific genomic sequences that are allowed to hybridize to tissue samples. Using probes targeting loci on 6p25 (RREB1), 6q23 (MYB), 6 centromere, and 11q13 (CCND1) for copy number changes, researchers found that using certain cutoff values permitted a test sensitivity from 82% to 94% and specificity from 90 to 98% [61–65]. The criteria for FISH positivity as provided by Gerami et al. include gain in RREB1 relative to CEP6 of at least 55%, gain in RREB1 greater than 29%, loss of MYB relative to CEP6 greater than 40%, and gain in CCND1 greater than 38% [62, 63]. These test criteria allowed for the correct identification of six out of six lesions with ambiguous pathology that later metastasized [62]. These criteria may have lower sensitivity and specificity in morphologically ambiguous melanocytic neoplasms, spitzoid neoplasms, and Spitz nevus (which may have tetraploidy, leading to false positives), so including probes for 8p24 (C-MYC) and 9p21 (CDKN2A) is proposed to increase the diagnostic utility of FISH [66].

Comparative genomic hybridization (CGH) can also aid in distinguishing nevi from melanoma based on chromosomal aberrations. Compared to melanomas, of which 96.2% had some form of chromosomal aberration, only 13% of benign nevi had aberrations [67]. Array-based CGH and single-nucleotide polymorphisms (SNP) arrays have been developed to increase resolution, reproducibility, and robustness of detecting these aberrations compared to traditional CGH [68–70]. With array-based CGH, the labeled tumor DNA is allowed to hybridize onto an array containing several loci and its signal intensity is compared to a reference normal DNA [71]. SNP arrays allow for the detection of smaller mutational changes that are missed by CGH arrays such as changes in allelic ratios and copy-neutral loss of heterozygosity [72].

There is generally high concordance between FISH and CGH, although there may be instances when one is preferred over the other. CGH has the advantage of covering vast regions of the genome and is therefore more likely to detect aberrations. FISH carries the advantage of requiring smaller amounts of specimen, lower purity because cells are visualized directly, less labor, and is typically quicker and of lower cost [71].

Analysis of genetic alterations and chromosomal aberrations allows for the identification of patterns beyond what we can gather from the clinic and histopathology. This is especially helpful for lesions that are ambiguous and difficult to diagnose, by aiding in making the final diagnosis, guide treatment decision-making, or increase the accuracy of prognosis. While no single test is definitive, these are tools that should be used to reinforce the histopathological diagnosis in consideration of the clinical context (Fig. 2.4).

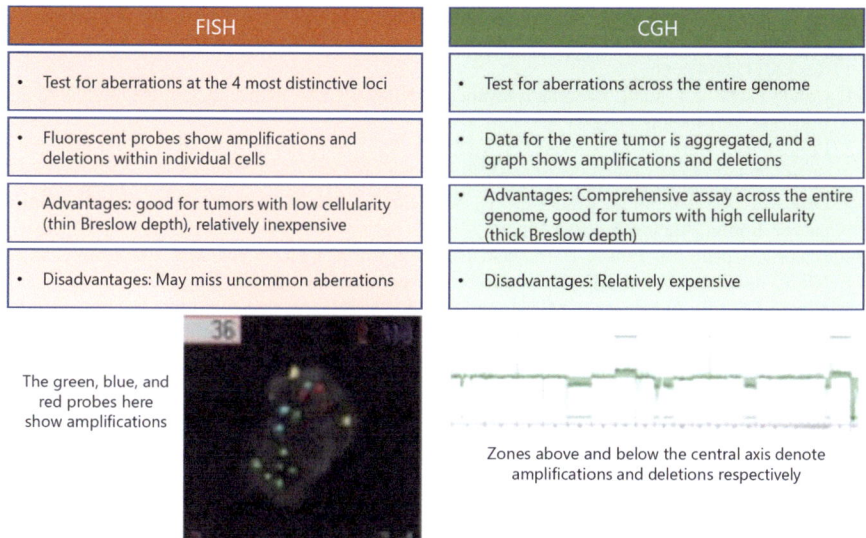

Fig. 2.4 Comparison of FISH and CGH Currently, melanocytic tumors can be tested using fluorescence in situ hybridization (FISH) or comparative genomic hybridization (CGH). Image courtesy of Jeff North, MD

References

1. Colebatch AJ, Scolyer RA. Trajectories of premalignancy during the journey from melanocyte to melanoma. Pathology (Phila). 2018;50(1):16–23.
2. Melamed RD, Aydin IT, Rajan GS, Phelps R, Silvers DN, Emmett KJ, et al. Genomic characterization of dysplastic nevi unveils implications for diagnosis of melanoma. J Invest Dermatol. 2017;137(4):905–9.
3. Erlich TH, Fisher DE. Pathways in melanoma development. G Ital Dermatol E Venereol. 2018;153(1):68–76.
4. Tsao H, Chin L, Garraway LA, Fisher DE. Melanoma: from mutations to medicine. Genes Dev. 2012;26(11):1131–55.
5. Lovly CM, Dahlman KB, Fohn LE, Su Z, Dias-Santagata D, Hicks DJ, et al. Routine multiplex mutational profiling of melanomas enables enrollment in genotype-driven therapeutic trials. PLoS One. 2012;7(4):e35309.
6. Rubinstein JC, Sznol M, Pavlick AC, Ariyan S, Cheng E, Bacchiocchi A, et al. Incidence of the V600K mutation among melanoma patients with BRAF mutations, and potential therapeutic response to the specific BRAF inhibitor PLX4032. J Transl Med. 2010;8:67.
7. Long GV, Menzies AM, Nagrial AM, Haydu LE, Hamilton AL, Mann GJ, et al. Prognostic and Clinicopathologic associations of oncogenic BRAF in metastatic melanoma. J Clin Oncol. 2011;29(10):1239–46.
8. Coricovac D, Dehelean C, Moaca E-A, Pinzaru I, Bratu T, Navolan D, et al. Cutaneous melanoma-a long road from experimental models to clinical outcome: a review. Int J Mol Sci. 2018;19(6):1566.
9. Saldanha G, Potter L, Daforno P, Pringle JH. Cutaneous melanoma subtypes show different BRAF and NRAS mutation frequencies. Clin Cancer Res. 2006;12(15):4499–505.

10. Devitt B, Liu W, Salemi R, Wolfe R, Kelly J, Tzen C-Y, et al. Clinical outcome and pathological features associated with NRAS mutation in cutaneous melanoma. Pigment Cell Melanoma Res. 2011;24(4):666–72.
11. Conde-Perez A, Larue L. Human relevance of NRAS/BRAF mouse melanoma models. Eur J Cell Biol. 2014;93(1–2):82–6.
12. Pollock PM, Harper UL, Hansen KS, Yudt LM, Stark M, Robbins CM, et al. High frequency of BRAF mutations in nevi. Nat Genet. 2003;33(1):19–20.
13. Leonardi GC, Accardi G, Monastero R, Nicoletti F, Libra M. Ageing: from inflammation to cancer. Immun Ageing A. 2018;15:1.
14. Bauer J, Curtin JA, Pinkel D, Bastian BC. Congenital melanocytic nevi frequently harbor NRAS mutations but no BRAF mutations. J Invest Dermatol. 2007;127(1):179–82.
15. Martín-Gorgojo A, Nagore E. Melanoma arising in a melanocytic nevus. Actas Dermosifiliogr. 2018;109(2):123–32.
16. Leonardi GC, Falzone L, Salemi R, Zanghì A, Spandidos DA, Mccubrey JA, et al. Cutaneous melanoma: from pathogenesis to therapy (review). Int J Oncol. 2018;52(4):1071–80.
17. Rawson RV, Scolyer RA. From Breslow to BRAF and immunotherapy: evolving concepts in melanoma pathogenesis and disease progression and their implications for changing management over the last 50 years. Hum Pathol. 2020;95:149–60.
18. Hodis E, Watson IR, Kryukov GV, Arold ST, Imielinski M, Theurillat J-P, et al. A landscape of driver mutations in melanoma. Cell. 2012;150(2):251–63.
19. Wu H, Goel V, Haluska FG. PTEN signaling pathways in melanoma. Oncogene. 2003;22(20):3113–22.
20. Soura E, Eliades PJ, Shannon K, Stratigos AJ, Tsao H. Hereditary melanoma: update on syndromes and management: genetics of familial atypical multiple mole melanoma syndrome. J Am Acad Dermatol. 2016;74(3):395–407. quiz 408–10
21. Gruis NA, van der Velden PA, Sandkuijl LA, Prins DE, Weaver-Feldhaus J, Kamb A, et al. Homozygotes for CDKN2 (p16) germline mutation in Dutch familial melanoma kindreds. Nat Genet. 1995;10(3):351–3.
22. Zuo L, Weger J, Yang Q, Goldstein AM, Tucker MA, Walker GJ, et al. Germline mutations in the p16INK4a binding domain of CDK4 in familial melanoma. Nat Genet. 1996;12(1):97–9.
23. Gast A, Scherer D, Chen B, Bloethner S, Melchert S, Sucker A, et al. Somatic alterations in the melanoma genome: a high-resolution array-based comparative genomic hybridization study. Genes Chromosom Cancer. 2010;49(8):733–45.
24. Maertens O, Johnson B, Hollstein P, Frederick DT, Cooper ZA, Messiaen L, et al. Elucidating distinct roles for NF1 in melanomagenesis. Cancer Discov. 2013;3(3):338–49.
25. Nissan MH, Pratilas CA, Jones AM, Ramirez R, Won H, Liu C, et al. Loss of NF1 in cutaneous melanoma is associated with RAS activation and MEK dependence. Cancer Res. 2014;74(8):2340–50.
26. Beadling C, Jacobson-Dunlop E, Hodi FS, Le C, Warrick A, Patterson J, et al. KIT gene mutations and copy number in melanoma subtypes. Clin Cancer Res. 2008;14(21):6821–8.
27. Handolias D, Salemi R, Murray W, Tan A, Liu W, Viros A, et al. Mutations in KIT occur at low frequency in melanomas arising from anatomical sites associated with chronic and intermittent sun exposure. Pigment Cell Melanoma Res. 2010;23(2):210–5.
28. Merkel EA, Gerami P. Malignant melanoma of sun-protected sites: a review of clinical, histological, and molecular features. Lab Investig. 2017;97(6):630–5.
29. Huang FW, Hodis E, Xu MJ, Kryukov GV, Chin L, Garraway LA. Highly recurrent TERT promoter mutations in human melanoma. Science. 2013;339(6122):957–9.
30. Horn S, Figl A, Rachakonda PS, Fischer C, Sucker A, Gast A, et al. TERT promoter mutations in familial and sporadic melanoma. Science. 2013;339(6122):959–61.
31. Del Bianco P, Stagni C, Giunco S, Fabozzi A, Elefanti L, Pellegrini S, et al. TERT promoter mutations differently correlate with the clinical outcome of MAPK inhibitor-treated melanoma patients. Cancers. 2020;12(4):946.
32. Shtivelman E, Davies MA, Hwu P, Yang J, Lotem M, Oren M, et al. Pathways and therapeutic targets in melanoma. Oncotarget. 2014;5(7):1701–52.

33. Polsky D, Bastian BC, Hazan C, Melzer K, Pack J, Houghton A, et al. HDM2 protein overexpression, but not gene amplification, is related to tumorigenesis of cutaneous melanoma. Cancer Res. 2001;61(20):7642–6.
34. Gembarska A, Luciani F, Fedele C, Russell EA, Dewaele M, Villar S, et al. MDM4 is a key therapeutic target in cutaneous melanoma. Nat Med. 2012;18(8):1239–47.
35. Matin RN, Chikh A, Chong SLP, Mesher D, Graf M. Sanza' P, et al. p63 is an alternative p53 repressor in melanoma that confers chemoresistance and a poor prognosis. J Exp Med. 2013;210(3):581–603.
36. Bergamaschi D, Samuels Y, Sullivan A, Zvelebil M, Breyssens H, Bisso A, et al. iASPP preferentially binds p53 proline-rich region and modulates apoptotic function of codon 72-polymorphic p53. Nat Genet. 2006;38(10):1133–41.
37. Van Raamsdonk CD, Griewank KG, Crosby MB, Garrido MC, Vemula S, Wiesner T, et al. Mutations in GNA11 in uveal melanoma. N Engl J Med. 2010;363(23):2191–9.
38. Cheng L, Lopez-Beltran A, Massari F, MacLennan GT, Montironi R. Molecular testing for BRAF mutations to inform melanoma treatment decisions: a move toward precision medicine. Mod Pathol. 2018;31(1):24–38.
39. Health C for D and R. List of Cleared or Approved Companion Diagnostic Devices (In Vitro and Imaging Tools). FDA [Internet]. 2020 Sep 10 [cited 2020 Sep 25]. https://www.fda.gov/medical-devices/vitro-diagnostics/list-cleared-or-approved-companion-diagnostic-devices-vitro-and-imaging-tools.
40. Gatter K. FDA oversight of laboratory-developed tests: where are we now? Arch Pathol Lab Med. 2017;141(6):746–8.
41. FDA Moves to Regulate Thousands of Diagnostic Tests [Internet]. AJMC. [cited 2020 Sep 25]. https://www.ajmc.com/view/fda-moves-to-regulate-thousands-of-diagnostic-tests.
42. Hodi FS, O'Day SJ, McDermott DF, Weber RW, Sosman JA, Haanen JB, et al. Improved survival with ipilimumab in patients with metastatic melanoma. N Engl J Med. 2010;363(8):711–23.
43. Ribas A, Puzanov I, Dummer R, Schadendorf D, Hamid O, Robert C, et al. Pembrolizumab versus investigator-choice chemotherapy for ipilimumab-refractory melanoma (KEYNOTE-002): a randomised, controlled, phase 2 trial. Lancet Oncol. 2015;16(8):908–18.
44. Weber JS, D'Angelo SP, Minor D, Hodi FS, Gutzmer R, Neyns B, et al. Nivolumab versus chemotherapy in patients with advanced melanoma who progressed after anti-CTLA-4 treatment (CheckMate 037): a randomised, controlled, open-label, phase 3 trial. Lancet Oncol. 2015;16(4):375–84.
45. Su F, Viros A, Milagre C, Trunzer K, Bollag G, Spleiss O, et al. RAS mutations in cutaneous squamous-cell carcinomas in patients treated with BRAF inhibitors. N Engl J Med. 2012;366(3):207–15.
46. Robert C, Karaszewska B, Schachter J, Rutkowski P, Mackiewicz A, Stroiakovski D, et al. Improved overall survival in melanoma with combined Dabrafenib and Trametinib. N Engl J Med. 2015;372(1):30–9.
47. Long GV, Stroyakovskiy D, Gogas H, Levchenko E, de Braud F, Larkin J, et al. Dabrafenib and trametinib versus dabrafenib and placebo for Val600 BRAF-mutant melanoma: a multicentre, double-blind, phase 3 randomised controlled trial. Lancet Lond Engl. 2015;386(9992):444–51.
48. Ascierto PA, McArthur GA, Dréno B, Atkinson V, Liszkay G, Giacomo AMD, et al. Cobimetinib combined with vemurafenib in advanced BRAFV600-mutant melanoma (coBRIM): updated efficacy results from a randomised, double-blind, phase 3 trial. Lancet Oncol. 2016;17(9):1248–60.
49. Daud A, Gill J, Kamra S, Chen L, Ahuja A. Indirect treatment comparison of dabrafenib plus trametinib versus vemurafenib plus cobimetinib in previously untreated metastatic melanoma patients. J Hematol Oncol. 2017;10(1):3.
50. Raskin L, Ludgate M, Iyer RK, Ackley TE, Bradford CR, Johnson TM, et al. Copy number variations and clinical outcome in atypical spitz tumors. Am J Surg Pathol. 2011;35(2):243–52.
51. Coit DG, Thompson JA, Albertini MR, Barker C, Carson WE, Contreras C, et al. Cutaneous melanoma, version 2.2019, NCCN clinical practice guidelines in oncology. J Natl Compr Cancer Netw. 2019;17(4):367–402.

52. Guo J, Si L, Kong Y, Flaherty KT, Xu X, Zhu Y, et al. Phase II, open-label, single-arm trial of imatinib mesylate in patients with metastatic melanoma harboring c-kit mutation or amplification. J Clin Oncol. 2011;29(21):2904–9.
53. Carvajal RD, Antonescu CR, Wolchok JD, Chapman PB, Roman R-A, Teitcher J, et al. KIT as a therapeutic target in metastatic melanoma. JAMA. 2011;305(22):2327–34.
54. Wei X, Mao L, Chi Z, Sheng X, Cui C, Kong Y, et al. Efficacy evaluation of Imatinib for the treatment of melanoma: evidence from a retrospective study. Oncol Res. 2019;27(4):495–501.
55. Hodi FS, Corless CL, Giobbie-Hurder A, Fletcher JA, Zhu M, Marino-Enriquez A, et al. Imatinib for melanomas harboring mutationally activated or amplified KIT arising on mucosal, acral, and chronically sun-damaged skin. J Clin Oncol. 2013;31(26):3182–90.
56. Meng D, Carvajal RD. KIT as an oncogenic driver in melanoma: an update on clinical development. Am J Clin Dermatol. 2019 Jun 1;20(3):315–23.
57. Peng W, Chen JQ, Liu C, Malu S, Creasy C, Tetzlaff MT, et al. Loss of PTEN promotes resistance to T cell-mediated immunotherapy. Cancer Discov. 2016;6(2):202–16.
58. Nathanson KL, Martin A-M, Wubbenhorst B, Greshock J, Letrero R, D'Andrea K, et al. Tumor genetic analyses of patients with metastatic melanoma treated with the BRAF inhibitor Dabrafenib (GSK2118436). Clin Cancer Res. 2013;19(17):4868–78.
59. Dijk MCRFV, Aben KKH, Hees FV, Klaasen A, Blokx WAM, Kiemeney LALM, et al. Expert review remains important in the histopathological diagnosis of cutaneous melanocytic lesions. Histopathology. 2008;52(2):139–46.
60. Lodha S, Saggar S, Celebi JT, Silvers DN. Discordance in the histopathologic diagnosis of difficult melanocytic neoplasms in the clinical setting. J Cutan Pathol. 2008;35(4):349–52.
61. Busam KJ. Molecular pathology of melanocytic tumors. Semin Diagn Pathol. 2013;30(4):362–74.
62. Gerami P, Jewell SS, Morrison LE, Blondin B, Schulz J, Ruffalo T, et al. Fluorescence in situ hybridization (FISH) as an ancillary diagnostic tool in the diagnosis of melanoma. Am J Surg Pathol. 2009;33(8):1146–56.
63. Vergier B, Prochazkova-Carlotti M, de la Fouchardière A, Cerroni L, Massi D, De Giorgi V, et al. Fluorescence in situ hybridization, a diagnostic aid in ambiguous melanocytic tumors: European study of 113 cases. Mod Pathol. 2011;24(5):613–23.
64. Moore MW, Gasparini R. FISH as an effective diagnostic tool for the management of challenging melanocytic lesions. Diagn Pathol. 2011;6:76.
65. Hossain D, Qian J, Adupe J, Drewnowska K, Bostwick DG. Differentiation of melanoma and benign nevi by fluorescence in-situ hybridization. Melanoma Res. 2011;21(5):426–30.
66. Ferrara G, De Vanna AC. Fluorescence in situ hybridization for melanoma diagnosis: a review and a reappraisal. Am J Dermatopathol. 2016;38(4):253–69.
67. Bastian BC, Olshen AB, LeBoit PE, Pinkel D. Classifying melanocytic tumors based on DNA copy number changes. Am J Pathol. 2003;163(5):1765–70.
68. Pinkel D, Segraves R, Sudar D, Clark S, Poole I, Kowbel D, et al. High resolution analysis of DNA copy number variation using comparative genomic hybridization to microarrays. Nat Genet. 1998;20(2):207–11.
69. Pollack JR, Perou CM, Alizadeh AA, Eisen MB, Pergamenschikov A, Williams CF, et al. Genome-wide analysis of DNA copy-number changes using cDNA microarrays. Nat Genet. 1999;23(1):41–6.
70. Solinas-Toldo S, Lampel S, Stilgenbauer S, Nickolenko J, Benner A, Döhner H, et al. Matrix-based comparative genomic hybridization: biochips to screen for genomic imbalances. Genes Chromosomes Cancer. 1997;20(4):399–407.
71. Miedema J, Andea AA. Through the looking glass and what you find there: making sense of comparative genomic hybridization and fluorescence in situ hybridization for melanoma diagnosis. Mod Pathol. 2020;33(7):1318–30.
72. Jacobs S, Thompson ER, Nannya Y, Yamamoto G, Pillai R, Ogawa S, et al. Genome-wide, high-resolution detection of copy number, loss of heterozygosity, and genotypes from formalin-fixed, paraffin-embedded tumor tissue using microarrays. Cancer Res. 2007;67(6):2544–51.

Familial Melanoma 3

Roughly 10% of melanomas develop in individuals with one or more first-degree relatives who also have melanoma [1]. Although there are no absolute features for familial melanoma, some patterns include a younger age at diagnosis, better survival, smaller lesions, and multiple primary lesions [2–4]. Situations to suspect an inherited predisposing gene mutation are in an individual who has any one family member with more than one melanoma or pancreatic cancer, several members on one side of the family diagnosed with melanoma, a personal history of two or more Spitz nevi, or a personal history of three or more melanomas [5, 6]. In a study of data from the Swedish Family-Cancer Database, 92% of melanoma patients with a family history had just one other affected family member, 7.3% had two other affected family members, and 0.6% had three or more other affected family members [7]. An individual's relative risk for developing melanoma corresponded with the number of affected family members: 2.42 for one relative, 6.49 for two relatives, and 8.30 for three or more relatives [7]. This relationship can be due to factors such as shared phenotypic traits, sun exposure patterns, or germline mutations.

Genetic Mutations

The most common locus with germline mutations associated with increased risk of developing melanoma is CDKN2A, of which there are at least 67 variants [8]. Mutations in the CDKN2A locus account for 25–40% of melanoma clustering in families [9, 10]. Among families with at least three confirmed individuals with melanoma, the frequency of CDKN2A mutations was found to vary by geographic region, at 20% of families in Australia and 45% of families in North America to 57% of families in Europe [11]. The penetrance of melanoma by 50 years of age in CDKN2A mutation carriers also varies by geographic location, which reaches 0.13 in Europe, 0.50 in the United States, and 0.32 in Australia [12]. The lifetime penetrance (by 80 years of age) increases to 0.58 in Europe, 0.76 in the United States, and 0.91 in Australia [11, 12].

The CDKN2A locus encodes two tumor suppressor proteins, p16INK4A and p14ARF, via alternative splicing. The p16 inhibitor of cyclin-dependent kinase 4 (p16INK4A) inhibits CDK4 and CDK6, leading to hypo-phosphorylation of RB that prevents E2F from allowing cell cycle progression from the G1 phase to the S phase. p14ARF inhibits MDM2 to promote the stability of p53, which carries antiproliferative and apoptotic effects [13]. CDKN2A and less so CDK4 have been best recognized as familial melanoma genes.

Mutations in CDK4, BAP1, TERT, POT1, ACD, TERF2IP, and MIP are far less likely than CDKN2A, contributing to a combined 10% of familial clustering of melanoma [14]. Seventeen families have a known mutation in the CDK4 gene, in which an activating mutation increases the likelihood of melanoma through a similar effect as p16INK4A mutations [15]. CDK4 interacts with cyclin D to phosphorylate Rb, which frees the E2F transcription factors to allow transcription of proteins to initiate the S phase.

Other gene mutations have been found to have high-penetrance associations with cancers such as melanoma and pancreatic cancer [16]. Protection of telomeres 1 (POT1) and TERT are two genes that are associated with familial melanoma when mutated [17]. Both serve a role in preventing chromosomal loss with cell replications; therefore aberrant activity in their proteins removes one of the natural cellular limits of proliferation. Germline variants of POT1 were found in almost 4% of familial melanoma pedigrees that had wild-type CDKN2A and CDK4 [17]. BAP1, ACD, and TERF2IP are also genes that, when mutated, are found to be associated with a high penetrance of melanoma [18].

Some genes found to have intermediate penetrance of increased melanoma risk are MC1R and MITF [14, 19, 20]. MC1R is the human melanocortin-1 receptor, whose ligand is melanocyte-stimulating hormone, and is a key controller of pigmentation [20]. Mutations in MC1R are associated with some phenotypes such as red hair, fair skin, and increased risk of skin cancers including melanoma [19, 21]. CDKN2A mutation carriers with one MC1R variant have a higher risk of melanoma than those who carry just a CDKN2A mutation and no MC1R mutation (OR = 2.2) [19]. The microphthalmia-associated transcription factor (MITF) stimulates hypoxia-inducible factor 1A (HIF1A) and can exhibit a germline missense mutation (E318K) in which carriers exhibit a fivefold increase in developing melanoma, renal cell carcinoma, or both [22]. A few other genes associated with melanoma in families found through whole-exome sequencing include ATM, CDKN2B, TYR, CDKAL1, PRKDC, MLLT4, PLCE1, MAP2K2, IL1RN, and ATR [23].

Genetic Testing and Counseling

Suspecting familial melanoma early and identifying a mutation such as CDKN2A, which is associated with a relatively high penetrance of melanoma, can allow patients and their families to make better informed decisions, but genetic testing has been controversial in clinical practice. Nearly 50% of familial melanomas currently cannot be attributed to any known inherited gene mutation [24]. The possible genes

Table 3.1 The rule of 2s and rule of 3s as minimum criteria for genetic testing of melanoma susceptibility

Rule of 2s	Rule of 3s
Two primary melanomas in an individual (or) Two cases of melanoma or pancreatic cancer, with at least one invasive melanoma, among first-or second-degree relatives on the same side of the family	Three primary melanomas in an individual (or) Three cases of melanoma or pancreatic cancer, with at least one invasive melanoma, among first-or second-degree relatives on the same side of the family

Data from Leachman SA et al. [25]

and alleles that might be involved are variable, and for many genes, there are a limited number of cases on which to base penetrance estimates. Some guidelines have been proposed to aid in determining the criteria for genetic testing, taking into consideration the general incidence rate of melanoma in which an individual has lived. This adjusts for the influence of environment, such that individuals who develop melanoma in a low incidence region have a greater likelihood of carrying an inherited predisposing mutation. The rule of 2s applies to areas with low incidence of melanoma such as Southern Europe, while the rule of 3s applies to areas with moderate to high incidence of melanoma such as the United States and Northern Europe, and a rule of 4s has been proposed for areas with very high incidence such as Australia [14, 25, 26]. Clinicians should note that these rules do not consider other factors such as age of diagnosis, family size, occupation, and sun-protective behaviors of the patient or their relatives with melanoma (Table 3.1).

Even without genetic testing or after receiving a negative result, individuals with a personal or family history of melanoma are still at increased risk of developing melanoma [27, 28]. These individuals are encouraged to undergo total body skin examination by a healthcare provider with the aid of full body photography or dermoscopy at minimum yearly. Those at high risk should be educated on the warning signs of melanoma, taught skin self-examination techniques, and instructed about practicing measures of sun protection. First-degree relatives of an individual diagnosed with melanoma may also be at increased risk for other cancers such as prostate, breast, and colon cancers, non-Hodgkin's lymphoma, and multiple myeloma [29]. Understanding the genetic basis of familial cancers such as melanoma has come a long way, but there are still many unknowns that make risk determination far from definitive. Improvement in the ability to identifying individuals at risk and their level of risk likely requires continued progress in identifying familial patterns of cancer as well as in the understanding and testability of genetics and other inherited features such as epigenetics.

References

1. Goldstein AM, Tucker MA. Genetic epidemiology of cutaneous melanoma: a global perspective. Arch Dermatol. 2001;137(11):1493–6.
2. Berwick M, Erdei E, Hay J. Melanoma epidemiology and public health. Dermatol Clin. 2009;27(2):205–14.

3. Kopf AW, Hellman LJ, Rogers GS, Gross DF, Rigel DS, Friedman RJ, et al. Familial malignant melanoma. JAMA. 1986;256(14):1915–9.
4. Taylor NJ, Mitra N, Qian L, Avril M-F, Bishop DT, Bressac-de Paillerets B, et al. Estimating CDKN2A mutation carrier probability among global familial melanoma cases using GenoMELPREDICT. J Am Acad Dermatol. 2019;81(2):386–94.
5. Schadendorf D, van Akkooi ACJ, Berking C, Griewank KG, Gutzmer R, Hauschild A, et al. Melanoma. Lancet. 2018;392(10151):971–84.
6. Swetter SM, Tsao H, Bichakjian CK, Curiel-Lewandrowski C, Elder DE, Gershenwald JE, et al. Guidelines of care for the management of primary cutaneous melanoma. J Am Acad Dermatol. 2019;80(1):208–50.
7. Frank C, Sundquist J, Hemminki A, Hemminki K. Risk of other cancers in families with melanoma: novel familial links. Sci Rep. 2017;7(1):42601.
8. Goldstein AM. Familial melanoma, pancreatic cancer and germline CDKN2A mutations. Hum Mutat. 2004;23(6):630.
9. Hayward NK. Genetics of melanoma predisposition. Oncogene. 2003;22(20):3053–62.
10. Potrony M, Badenas C, Aguilera P, Puig-Butille JA, Carrera C, Malvehy J, et al. Update in genetic susceptibility in melanoma. Ann Transl Med. 2015;3(15):210.
11. Goldstein AM, Chan M, Harland M, Hayward NK, Demenais F, Bishop DT, et al. Features associated with germline CDKN2A mutations: a GenoMEL study of melanoma-prone families from three continents. J Med Genet. 2007;44(2):99–106.
12. Bishop DT, Demenais F, Goldstein AM, Bergman W, Bishop JN, Bressac-de Paillerets B, et al. Geographical variation in the penetrance of CDKN2A mutations for melanoma. J Natl Cancer Inst. 2002;94(12):894–903.
13. Zhang Y, Xiong Y, Yarbrough WG. ARF promotes MDM2 degradation and stabilizes p53: ARF-INK4a locus deletion impairs both the Rb and p53 tumor suppression pathways. Cell. 1998;92(6):725–34.
14. Rossi M, Pellegrini C, Cardelli L, Ciciarelli V, Di Nardo L, Fargnoli MC. Familial melanoma: diagnostic and management implications. Dermatol Pract Concept. 2019;9(1):10–6.
15. Puntervoll HE, Yang XR, Vetti HH, Bachmann IM, Avril MF, Benfodda M, et al. Melanoma prone families with CDK4 germline mutation: phenotypic profile and associations with MC1R variants. J Med Genet. 2013;50(4):264–70.
16. Newton-Bishop J, Bishop D, Harland M. Melanoma genomics. Acta Derm Venereol. 2020;100(11):adv00138.
17. Robles-Espinoza CD, Harland M, Ramsay AJ, Aoude LG, Quesada V, Ding Z, et al. POT1 loss-of-function variants predispose to familial melanoma. Nat Genet. 2014;46(5):478–81.
18. Read J, Wadt KAW, Hayward NK. Melanoma genetics. J Med Genet. 2016;53(1):1–14.
19. Fargnoli MC, Gandini S, Peris K, Maisonneuve P, Raimondi S. MC1R variants increase melanoma risk in families with CDKN2A mutations: a meta-analysis. Eur J Cancer Oxf Engl. 2010;46(8):1413–20.
20. Pasquali E, García-Borrón JC, Fargnoli MC, Gandini S, Maisonneuve P, Bagnardi V, et al. MC1R variants increased the risk of sporadic cutaneous melanoma in darker-pigmented caucasians: a pooled-analysis from the M-SKIP project. Int J Cancer. 2015;136(3):618–31.
21. Beaumont KA, Shekar SL, Newton RA, James MR, Stow JL, Duffy DL, et al. Receptor function, dominant negative activity and phenotype correlations for MC1R variant alleles. Hum Mol Genet. 2007;16(18):2249–60.
22. Bertolotto C, Lesueur F, Giuliano S, Strub T, de Lichy M, Bille K, et al. A SUMOylation-defective MITF germline mutation predisposes to melanoma and renal carcinoma. Nature. 2011;480(7375):94–8.
23. Yepes S, Tucker MA, Koka H, Xiao Y, Jones K, Vogt A, et al. Using whole-exome sequencing and protein interaction networks to prioritize candidate genes for germline cutaneous melanoma susceptibility. Sci Rep. 2020;10(1):17198.
24. Udayakumar D, Tsao H. Melanoma genetics: an update on risk-associated genes. Hematol Oncol Clin North Am. 2009;23(3):415–29. vii

References

25. Leachman SA, Carucci J, Kohlmann W, Banks KC, Asgari MM, Bergman W, et al. Selection criteria for genetic assessment of patients with familial melanoma. J Am Acad Dermatol. 2009;61(4):677.e1–14.
26. Delaunay J, Martin L, Bressac-de Paillerets B, Duru G, Ingster O, Thomas L. Improvement of genetic testing for cutaneous melanoma in countries with low to moderate incidence. JAMA Dermatol. 2017;153(11):1122–9.
27. Goggins WB, Tsao H. A population-based analysis of risk factors for a second primary cutaneous melanoma among melanoma survivors. Cancer. 2003;97(3):639–43.
28. Badenas C, Aguilera P, Puig-Butillé JA, Carrera C, Malvehy J, Puig S. Genetic counselling in melanoma. Dermatol Ther. 2012;25(5):397–402.
29. Larson AA, Leachman SA, Eliason MJ, Cannon-Albright LA. Population-based assessment of non-melanoma cancer risk in relatives of cutaneous melanoma probands. J Invest Dermatol. 2007;127(1):183–8.

Treatment for Stages I–III

Stage 0 Treatment

Wide Local Excision [1–7]

The surgeon removes the rest of the tumor, including the biopsy site, as well as a surgical margin (a surrounding area of normal-appearing skin and the underlying subcutaneous tissue), to ensure the whole tumor has been removed. Margins taken: At least 0.5-cm margins in all directions (less than 0.25 in.).

Disease-free survival 5 years after treatment: 98% [8, 9]

Stage IA Treatment

Wide Local Excision

Treatment is consistent with that of Stage 0, but with margins of at least 1-cm margin in all directions (less than 0.5 in.).

Melanoma-specific survival 5 years after treatment: 99% [10]

Stage IB–II Treatment

Wide Local Excision and Sentinel Lymph Node (SLN) Biopsy

In addition to wide local excision, a SLN biopsy can be performed to provide additional prognostic data by determining if any malignant cells have spread to nearby nodes. The sentinel node is the first lymph node to receive drainage from the primary tumor and the site where melanomas commonly spread to first. SLN biopsy is most accurate when the lymph channels around the primary melanoma have not been disturbed by a prior wide excision. Therefore, in general, the SLN biopsy and wide excision are done during the same surgery, with the biopsy first.

SLN biopsy is recommended starting with Stage IB (<1.0 mm with ulceration or 0.8–2.0 mm without) as both Breslow thickness and ulceration are correlated with SLN positivity and nodal recurrence [11]. In several large clinical trials and meta-analyses, nodal metastases were uncommon in patients with melanoma primary lesions under 1 mm thick, with positive nodes seen in only 1–5.6% of patients [9, 12, 13]. The incidences of nodal metastases in patients with 1–2 mm deep and 2–4 mm deep primary lesions were 15% and 30%, respectively. In contrast, thick lesions with Breslow depths greater than 4 mm were associated with high rates of nodal metastases with estimates ranging from 35.5 to 45% [9, 12, 13].

To find the sentinel lymph node(s), the doctor injects a small amount of a radioactive solution (or a blue dye) into the area of the melanoma. After an hour or so, the doctor checks for radioactivity (or dye) in the lymph nodes areas near the tumor. For each area found, a small incision is made to remove the node for further examination by a pathologist. A SLN biopsy is considered positive if there are signs of melanoma in any of the examined nodes and negative otherwise. For a negative biopsy, no further treatment is required at the time because it is very unlikely the melanoma would have spread beyond the sentinel node. If melanoma cells are found and the biopsy is positive, treatment is consistent with that of Stage III disease discussed below.

If a lymph node near a melanoma is abnormally large, a sentinel node biopsy may not be needed. Instead, the enlarged node is simply biopsied.

See Table 4.1 for survival data in regard to sentinel node results [8–10, 14, 15].

- Melanoma-specific survival 5 years after treatment in Stage IB: 97% [10].
- Melanoma-specific survival 5 years after treatment in Stage IIA: 94% [10].
- Melanoma-specific survival 5 years after treatment in Stage IIB: 65% [10].
- Melanoma-specific survival 5 years after treatment in Stage IIC: 45% [10].

Table 4.1 Survival data in regard to sentinel node results [8–10, 14, 15]

	+SLN	−SLN
5y disease-free survival	53%	83%
5y melanoma-specific survival	72%	90%

Stage III Treatment

Baseline Imaging, Primary Treatment, and Adjuvant Treatment and/or Observation

For patients with surgically removable or resectable disease, primary treatment consists of wide excision of the primary tumor and a choice between further lymph node dissection or surveillance. In the past, lymph node dissection, which involved the removal of the remaining lymph nodes in an area, would be recommended as part of primary treatment if there was evidence that the melanoma had spread to nearby lymph nodes. If the melanoma was found by SLN biopsy, this is called a complete lymph node dissection (CLND). If the melanoma was found because of visibly enlarged lymph nodes, this is called a therapeutic lymph node dissection (TLND). The goal of the surgery is to prevent further spread of the disease in the body through the lymphatic system. However, since the results of two landmark trials (DeCOG-SLT and MSLT-II) demonstrated no increase in survival benefit for such surgery, nodal basin ultrasound surveillance can be considered over surgery especially in patients with low tumor burden [16, 17]. CLND/TLND can still be discussed with patients for therapeutic value or to better control regional disease if it outweighs the potential morbidities of the procedure.

If a patient has already been diagnosed with Stage III melanoma, a sentinel lymph node biopsy is typically recommended only for patients where it is suspected that there might be melanoma in another lymph node basin.

After any initial surgical procedures, systemic adjuvant therapy can be recommended to the patient for resectable Stage III melanoma in addition to observation. Systemic therapies travel throughout the bloodstream to target any remaining cancer cells throughout the body. Current regimens include the checkpoint inhibitors nivolumab and pembrolizumab (targets PD-1) and a targeted combination therapy dabrafenib/trametinib (targets BRAF/MEK). When discussing therapy options, it is important to consider factors like the risk of disease recurrence and the potential adverse effects of therapy.

Of the adjuvant therapy options, nivolumab or pembrolizumab is equally preferred for resected Stage IIIB/IIIC regardless of BRAF mutation [18, 19]. The safety profiles of these therapies are acceptable with fatigue, diarrhea, and pruritus as most common adverse events. Occurrence of high-grade (grade 3 or 4) adverse events is low and was observed to be about 14% in clinical trials [19, 20]. An alternative option for BRAF-mutated disease is combination dabrafenib/trametinib therapy, which results in quick initial response in most patients followed by resistance to treatment and recurrence with a 9.4-month median progression-free survival [21, 22]. Such therapy may be preferred if a patient is unsuited for immunotherapy (e.g., has autoimmune disease or on immunosuppressive drugs) or unable to withstand the potential toxicities of alternatives.

For patients with surgically unremovable or unresectable disease, primary treatment consists of a choice among local/regional and systemic therapies similar to that of Stage IV disease, which are discussed in Chaps. 5 and 6, respectively. Adjuvant therapies include the systemic options described above, radiation therapy, and observation.

- Melanoma-specific survival 5 years after treatment in Stage IIIA: 93% [10].
- Melanoma-specific survival 5 years after treatment in Stage IIIB: 83% [10].
- Melanoma-specific survival 5 years after treatment in Stage IIIC: 69% [10].
- Melanoma-specific survival 5 years after treatment in Stage IIID: 32% [10].

References

1. Veronesi U, Cascinelli N, Adamus J, Balch C, Bandiera D, Barchuk A, et al. Thin stage I primary cutaneous malignant melanoma. Comparison of excision with margins of 1 or 3 cm. N Engl J Med. 1988;318(18):1159–62.
2. Veronesi U, Cascinelli N. Narrow excision (1-cm margin). A safe procedure for thin cutaneous melanoma. Arch Surg. 1991;126(4):438–41.
3. Cohn-Cedermark G, Rutqvist LE, Andersson R, Breivald M, Ingvar C, Johansson H, et al. Long term results of a randomized study by the Swedish melanoma study group on 2-cm versus 5-cm resection margins for patients with cutaneous melanoma with a tumor thickness of 0.8-2.0 mm. Cancer. 2000;89(7):1495–501.
4. Khayat D, Rixe O, Martin G, Soubrane C, Banzet M, Bazex J-A, et al. Surgical margins in cutaneous melanoma (2 cm versus 5 cm for lesions measuring less than 2.1-mm thick). Cancer. 2003;97(8):1941–6.
5. Thomas JM, Newton-Bishop J, A'Hern R, Coombes G, Timmons M, Evans J, et al. Excision margins in high-risk malignant melanoma. N Engl J Med. 2004;350(8):757–66.
6. Heaton KM, Sussman JJ, Gershenwald JE, Lee JE, Reintgen DS, Mansfield PF, et al. Surgical margins and prognostic factors in patients with thick (>4mm) primary melanoma. Ann Surg Oncol. 1998;5(4):322–8.
7. Coit DG, Andtbacka R, Bichakjian CK, Dilawari RA, Dimaio D, Guild V, et al. Melanoma. J Natl Compr Cancer Netw. 2009;7(3):250–75.
8. Balch CM, Gershenwald JE, Soong S-J, Thompson JF, Atkins MB, Byrd DR, et al. Final version of 2009 AJCC melanoma staging and classification. J Clin Oncol. 2009;27(36):6199–206.
9. Algazi AP, Soon CW, Daud AI. Treatment of cutaneous melanoma: current approaches and future prospects. Cancer Manag Res. 2010;2:197–211.
10. Gershenwald JE, Scolyer RA, Hess KR, Sondak VK, Long GV, Ross MI, et al. Melanoma staging: evidence-based changes in the American joint committee on cancer eighth edition cancer staging manual. CA Cancer J Clin. 2017;67(6):472–92.
11. Yonick DV, Ballo RM, Kahn E, Dahiya M, Yao K, Godellas C, et al. Predictors of positive sentinel lymph node in thin melanoma. Am J Surg. 2011;201(3):324–8.
12. Lens MB, Dawes M, Newton-Bishop JA, Goodacre T. Tumour thickness as a predictor of occult lymph node metastases in patients with stage I and II melanoma undergoing sentinel lymph node biopsy. Br J Surg. 2002;89(10):1223–7.
13. Warycha MA, Zakrzewski J, Ni Q, Shapiro RL, Berman RS, Pavlick AC, et al. Meta-analysis of sentinel lymph node positivity in thin melanoma. Cancer. 2009;115(4):869–79.
14. Morton DL, Thompson JF, Cochran AJ, Mozzillo N, Elashoff R, Essner R, et al. Sentinel-node biopsy or nodal observation in melanoma. N Engl J Med. 2006;355(13):1307–17.

References

15. van Akkooi ACJ, Rutkowski P, van der Ploeg IM, Voit C, Robert C, Hoekstra HJ, et al. 9302 Excellent long-term survival of patients with minimal sentinel node tumor burden (<0.1 mm) according to Rotterdam criteria: a study of the EORTC melanoma group. Eur J Cancer Suppl. 2009;7(2):576–7.
16. Leiter U, Stadler R, Mauch C, Hohenberger W, Brockmeyer NH, Berking C, et al. Final analysis of DeCOG-SLT trial: no survival benefit for complete lymph node dissection in patients with melanoma with positive sentinel node. J Clin Oncol. 2019;37(32):3000–8.
17. Faries MB, Thompson JF, Cochran AJ, Andtbacka RH, Mozzillo N, Zager JS, et al. Completion dissection or observation for sentinel-node metastasis in melanoma. N Engl J Med. 2017;376(23):2211–22.
18. Weber JS, Del Vecchio M, Mandala M, Gogas H, Arance AM, Dalle S, et al. Adjuvant nivolumab (NIVO) versus ipilimumab (IPI) in resected stage III/IV melanoma: 3-year efficacy and biomarker results from the phase III CheckMate 238 trial. Ann Oncol. 2019;30:v533–4.
19. Weber J, Mandala M, Del Vecchio M, Gogas HJ, Arance AM, Cowey CL, et al. Adjuvant nivolumab versus ipilimumab in resected stage III or IV melanoma. N Engl J Med. 2017;377:1824–35.
20. Eggermont AMM, Blank CU, Mandala M, Long GV, Atkinson V, Dalle S, et al. Adjuvant pembrolizumab versus placebo in resected stage III melanoma. N Engl J Med. 2018;378(19):1789–801.
21. Flaherty KT, Infante JR, Daud A, Gonzalez R, Kefford RF, Sosman J, et al. Combined BRAF and MEK inhibition in melanoma with BRAF V600 mutations. N Engl J Med. 2012;367(18):1694–703.
22. Kakadia S, Yarlagadda N, Awad R, Kundranda M, Niu J, Naraev B, et al. Mechanisms of resistance to BRAF and MEK inhibitors and clinical update of US Food and Drug Administration-approved targeted therapy in advanced melanoma. Onco Targets Ther. 2018;11:7095–107.

Treatment for Regionally Advanced and In-transit Melanoma

In-transit Melanoma

Melanoma invades local tissues and then spreads via lymphatics. Regionally advanced disease includes melanoma that has spread between the primary tumor site and the regional lymph node basin. When these metastases are located within 2 cm from the primary melanoma, they are referred to as satellite metastases, while those that are greater than 2 cm from the primary melanoma are classified as in-transit metastases [1]. In-transit metastases may develop in 2–13% of patients diagnosed with melanoma and are more likely in those with greater Breslow depth, presence of ulceration, positive sentinel lymph node status, and age greater than 50 [2, 3]. In-transit lesions may be pigmented or nonpigmented and can present as blisters or subcutaneous, dermal, or cutaneous nodules and can even be mistaken as rashes [4]. Approximately 30–75% of patients with in-transit disease will eventually develop metastases to the regional nodes or more distant organs [3]. The 8th edition of the AJCC staging manual assigns patients with in-transit disease a "c" designation within nodal stage (N1c, N2c, and N3c for 0, 1, and 2+ regional lymph nodes involved, respectively) [1].

Therapy Options

For in-transit melanoma metastases, the goal is generally to resect lesions that can be resected, as surgical resection with sufficient margins remains the first-line treatment [5]. The specimens should be sent for pathology confirmation. If in-transit lesions are confirmed, CT and/or PET scans with brain CT/MRI can be used to evaluate for distant metastases [6]. Patients with concurrent clinically evident distant metastatic should be treated with systemic therapy as described in Chap. 6. For in-transit disease, systemic immunotherapy and targeted therapy has led to these agents being used with varying success [7].

The rest of this chapter discusses treatments for regionally advanced melanoma when there are no distant metastases and resection cannot be done. When in-transit disease is confined to an extremity, regionally directed therapies allow for more focused treatment without subjecting the rest of the body to potential adverse events [8]. Intraarterial therapies such as isolated limb perfusion (ILP) and isolated limb infusion (ILI) use high concentrations of cytotoxic agents while avoiding systemic toxicity [9, 10]. Alternatively, intralesional injection therapy may be used in patients with unresectable in-transit disease, high disease burden, or increased frailty [2]. Whenever possible, eligible patients should be encouraged to participate in a clinical trial [11].

Isolated Limb Perfusion (ILP)

Hyperthermic isolated limb perfusion (HILP) is a procedure performed under general anesthesia in the operating room, where the major vessels of the limb affected by in-transit melanoma are surgically dissected and cannulated to create an isolated circuit. A tourniquet is applied proximally that excludes vessels from systemic circulation, and a cardiopulmonary bypass circuit is used to circulate chemotherapy that has been heated to 39–42 °C [9]. Across 22 studies, a total of 2018 HILPs showed a median overall response rate (ORR) of 90%, complete response (CR) rate of 58%, and 5-year overall survival (OS) of 37% [12].

The durability of the response to ILP is moderate, with the best responses in patients who have achieved CR. The most used agent is the chemotherapeutic agent melphalan, which attaches alkyl groups to purine nucleotides. In studies evaluating the use of melphalan alone, or with IFN or TNF-α, the overall median recurrence rate was roughly 40.5% [13]. Another study found that median time to recurrence was 10.5 months [14]. In a study of long-term remission rates with 120 HILPs with various cytotoxic agents in 111 patients performed, 69% achieved complete remission, and 34% of these patients maintained complete remission for a median follow-up duration of 199 months [15]. A similar study of 155 in-transit melanoma patients treated with HILP found 65% had complete remission and 20% had partial response within a median follow-up time of 16 months [16]. Prognostic factors for complete remission include multiple versus single perfusion schedule, absence of regional node involvement, and leg versus other tumor sites [17].

A few studies have investigated the addition of TNF-α to melphalan ILP. One systematic review found that over 12 studies with 556 perfusions, the combination yielded a median CR rate of 68.9% compared to 46.5% in patients treated with melphalan alone [14]. In a study in 100 consecutive ILPs with the combination of TNF-α and melphalan, ORR was 95%, with 69% CR and 26% partial response [18]. However, one phase III randomized trial found no benefit for the addition of TNF-α to HILP with melphalan and overall lower CR rates than in other studies (25% in the melphalan-alone arm and 26% in the melphalan + TNF-α arm) [19].

Despite decreased systemic toxicity, there can be regional toxicity in the limb treated with ILP. In a retrospective study of patients treated between 1978 and 1999, side effects of regional isolated perfusion with melphalan include lymphedema (28%), muscle atrophy or fibrosis (11%), limb malfunction (15%), neuropathy (4%), pain (8%), and recurrent infection (3%) [20–23]. One study of 69 ILP procedures found that 8 cases (12%) had short-term neutropenia with 3 of these patients requiring hospitalization due to sepsis, and 2 had compartment syndrome requiring fasciotomy [24].

Isolated Limb Infusion (ILI)

ILI is a treatment approach similar to isolated limb perfusion with the use of a tourniquet to isolate the extremity vasculature and infusion of agents such as melphalan with or without other agents like actinomycin D [25]. Unlike ILP, which involves complete dissection of the limb's main vessels, ILI uses high-flow catheters in the artery and vein placed percutaneously from the uninvolved limb, which are then advanced into the artery and vein of the involved limb.

The benefits of ILI include lower flow rates, for a shorter duration [5]. It is thought that efficacy of ILI despite lower amounts of chemotherapeutic agent used is due to ILI not involving blood perfusion of the limb, which creates a progressively hypoxic and acidotic environment that can potentially enhance cytotoxic effects. Small nonrandomized retrospective studies comparing ILI and ILP showed that ILP had superior CR rate (80% for HILP vs. 53% for ILI) but decreased OS (40 months for HILP vs. 46 months for ILI) [12, 26].

One prospective database study of 185 patients treated with ILI with melphalan between 1993 and 2007 found an overall response rate of 84%, a CR rate of 38%, and a partial response rate of 46% [27]. In a single-institution retrospective study of 205 ILI among 163 patients, OR was 59%, with median PFS of 14 months and OS of 56 months for a median follow-up duration of 22 months [28]. A larger, multinational, multicenter study of 687 patients with a single ILI for Stage 3B or 3C melanoma reported an ORR of 64%, a CR of 35%, and a median OS of 38 months over median follow-up duration of 47 months [29].

Although ILI may have lower overall response rates compared to HILP, the convenience and simplicity, along with decreased rate of limb morbidity, may make ILI preferable [23]. With the development of systemic immunotherapy, ongoing studies are investigating its use after ILI. One phase II study of ipilimumab following ILI found ORR of 85% at 3 months and PFS of 58% after 1 year [30]. The notable adverse effects of this sequence of treatment were primarily immune related and the rates of more serious adverse effects were comparable to those published for adjuvant ipilimumab alone [31]. The high early response rates of ILI may lead to further research combining regional therapies with systemic therapies.

Intralesional Therapy

An alternative for regionally advanced melanoma that is relatively isolated is injection of a therapeutic agent directly in the lesion to maximize efficacy while minimizing systemic adverse effects. Often, the intent is to elicit a local immune response against the tumor cells. Intralesional Bacille Calmette-Guerin (BCG) was historically used, but it had poor response rates and a significant adverse event profile. A pooled analysis of 15 intralesional BCG trials for Stage III melanoma found CR rates of 19%, partial response in 26%, and extended survival in 13%, but adverse events included anaphylactic reactions and fatal disseminated BCG infection [32]. Its clinical use is now limited.

Systemic IL-2 was a treatment that was commonly used after trials found a durable long-term survival in those that achieved CR [33, 34]. However, the response rate was generally poor at just 10–15%, with adverse effects resembling systemic inflammatory response syndrome (SIRS) [35]. Intralesional injections of IL-2 were tried to induce a more targeted effect. A single-institution retrospective review of 65 consecutive patients that received at least 4 cycles of intralesional IL-2 therapy between 2009 and 2019 found that the clinical CR (lesion no longer palpable) rate was 44.6%, and of these patients, 62% experienced a grade 1 adverse event such as erythema, swelling, or mild flu-like symptoms [36]. At a median follow-up of 27 months, PFS was 65.5% and clinical CR was 69.0% [36]. A systematic review of 6 observational trials including 2182 in-transit melanoma lesions among 140 patients found CR in 78% of treated lesions and in 50% of patients [37]. These studies demonstrate promising effects of intralesional IL-2 without significant systemic adverse effects, though there may be a burden of frequent injection and considerable cost.

PV-10 (rose bengal disodium) is a water-soluble xanthene dye shown in preclinical studies to preferentially enter melanoma cell lysosomes and induce a cytotoxic release of proteasomes while sparing normal cells [38]. A phase I trial of 26 target lesions in 11 patients showed CR rate of 36% and ORR of 48% [39]. A phase II trial of 80 patients with Stage III or IV refractory melanoma who received intralesional PV-10 in up to 20 lesions, four times over 16 weeks, then followed for 52 weeks found ORR of 51% and CR of 26% [40].

Talimogene laherparepvec (T-VEC) is an oncolytic viral therapy using genetically modified HSV-1 and is FDA approved for locoregionally advanced melanoma. Granulocyte-macrophage colony-stimulating factor (GM-CSF) stimulates tumor immunity and has been studied for the treatment of advanced melanoma [41, 42]. In T-VEC, the HSV-1 neurovirulence factor ICP34.5 is replaced with GM-CSF to enhance MHC class I presentation of tumor antigens [43]. The OPTiM randomized phase III trial compared intralesional T-VEC to subcutaneous GM-CSF in 249 patients and found that the viral delivery modality led to significantly higher ORR (40.5 vs. 2.3%, $p < 0.0001$) [44]. The combination of T-VEC with immunotherapy has also been studied recently. A phase II study involving 198 patients randomly assigned to T-VEC + ipilimumab or ipilimumab alone showed that the combination led to a higher ORR (39% vs. 18%) [45]. Ongoing studies are evaluating whether a similar benefit can be seen with combining oncolytic virotherapy with anti-PD-1 therapy [46, 47].

References

1. Gershenwald JE, Scolyer RA, Hess KR, Sondak VK, Long GV, Ross MI, et al. Melanoma staging: evidence-based changes in the American Joint Committee on Cancer eighth edition cancer staging manual. CA Cancer J Clin. 2017;67(6):472–92.
2. Perone JA, Farrow N, Tyler DS, Beasley GM. Contemporary approaches to in-transit melanoma. J Oncol Pract. 2018;14(5):292–300.
3. Pawlik TM, Ross MI, Thompson JF, Eggermont AMM, Gershenwald JE. The risk of in-transit melanoma metastasis depends on tumor biology and not the surgical approach to regional lymph nodes. J Clin Oncol. 2005;23(21):4588–90.
4. Speicher PJ, Meriwether CH, Tyler DS. Regional therapies for in-transit disease. Surg Oncol Clin N Am. 2015;24(2):309–22.
5. Nan Tie E, Henderson MA, Gyorki DE. Management of in-transit melanoma metastases: a review. ANZ J Surg. 2019;89(6):647–52.
6. Coit DG, Andtbacka R, Bichakjian CK, Dilawari RA, Dimaio D, Guild V, et al. Melanoma. J Natl Compr Cancer Netw. 2009;7(3):250–75.
7. Read RL, Thompson JF. Managing in-transit melanoma metastases in the new era of effective systemic therapies for melanoma. Expert Rev Clin Pharmacol. 2019;12(12):1107–19.
8. Pointer DT, Zager JS. Management of locoregionally advanced melanoma. Surg Clin North Am. 2020;100(1):109–25.
9. Patel A, Carr MJ, Sun J, Zager JS. In-transit metastatic cutaneous melanoma: current management and future directions. Clin Exp Metastasis. 2022;39(1):201–11.
10. Long GV, Hauschild A, Santinami M, Atkinson V, Mandalà M, Chiarion-Sileni V, et al. Adjuvant dabrafenib plus trametinib in stage III BRAF-mutated melanoma. N Engl J Med. 2017;377(19):1813–23.
11. Swetter SM, Thompson JA, Albertini MR, Barker CA, Baumgartner J, Boland G, et al. NCCN guidelines® insights: melanoma: cutaneous, version 2.2021: featured updates to the NCCN guidelines. J Natl Compr Cancer Netw. 2021;19(4):364–76.
12. Grünhagen DJ, Verhoef C. Isolated limb perfusion for stage III melanoma: does it still have a role in the present era of effective systemic therapy? Oncologia. 2016;30(12):1045–52.
13. Daud A, Algazi A, Soon C. Treatment of cutaneous melanoma: current approaches and future prospects. Cancer Manag Res. 2010;2:197–211.
14. Moreno-Ramirez D, de la Cruz-Merino L, Ferrandiz L, Villegas-Portero R, Nieto-Garcia A. Isolated limb perfusion for malignant melanoma: systematic review on effectiveness and safety. Oncologist. 2010;15(4):416–27.
15. Sanki A, Kam PCA, Thompson JF. Long-term results of hyperthermic, isolated limb perfusion for melanoma: a reflection of tumor biology. Ann Surg. 2007;245(4):591–6.
16. Olofsson R, Mattsson J, Lindnér P. Long-term follow-up of 163 consecutive patients treated with isolated limb perfusion for in-transit metastases of malignant melanoma. Int J Hyperth. 2013;29(6):551–7.
17. Klaase JM, Kroon BB, van Geel AN, Eggermont AM, Franklin HR, Hart AA. Prognostic factors for tumor response and limb recurrence-free interval in patients with advanced melanoma of the limbs treated with regional isolated perfusion with melphalan. Surgery. 1994;115(1):39–45.
18. Grünhagen DJ, Brunstein F, Graveland WJ, van Geel AN, de Wilt JHW, Eggermont AMM. One hundred consecutive isolated limb perfusions with TNF-α and melphalan in melanoma patients with multiple in-transit metastases. Ann Surg. 2004;240(6):939–48.

19. Cornett WR, McCall LM, Petersen RP, Ross MI, Briele HA, Noyes RD, et al. Randomized multicenter trial of hyperthermic isolated limb perfusion with melphalan alone compared with melphalan plus tumor necrosis factor: American College of Surgeons Oncology Group Trial Z0020. J Clin Oncol. 2006;24(25):4196–201.
20. Vrouenraets BC, Klaase JM, Kroon BB, van Geel BN, Eggermont AM, Franklin HR. Long-term morbidity after regional isolated perfusion with melphalan for melanoma of the limbs. The influence of acute regional toxic reactions. Arch Surg. 1995;130(1):43–7.
21. Santillan AA, Delman KA, Beasley GM, Mosca PJ, Hochwald SN, Grobmyer SR, et al. Predictive factors of regional toxicity and serum creatine phosphokinase levels after isolated limb infusion for melanoma: a multi-institutional analysis. Ann Surg Oncol. 2009;16(9):2570–8.
22. Möller MG, Lewis JM, Dessureault S, Zager JS. Toxicities associated with hyperthermic isolated limb perfusion and isolated limb infusion in the treatment of melanoma and sarcoma. Int J Hyperth. 2008;24(3):275–89.
23. Raymond AK, Beasley GM, Broadwater G, Augustine CK, Padussis JC, Turley R, et al. Current trends in regional therapy for melanoma: lessons learned from 225 regional chemotherapy treatments between 1995 and 2010 at a single institution. J Am Coll Surg. 2011;213(2):306–16.
24. Tulokas SKA, Kohtamäki LM, Mäkelä SP, Juteau S, Albäck A, Vikatmaa PJ, et al. Isolated limb perfusion with melphalan as treatment for regionally advanced melanoma of the limbs: results of 60 patients treated in Finland during 2007–2018. Melanoma Res. 2021;31(5):456–63.
25. Thompson JF, Kam PC, Waugh RC, Harman CR. Isolated limb infusion with cytotoxic agents: a simple alternative to isolated limb perfusion. Semin Surg Oncol. 1998;14(3):238–47.
26. Dossett LA, Ben-Shabat I, Olofsson Bagge R, Zager JS. Clinical response and regional toxicity following isolated limb infusion compared with isolated limb perfusion for in-transit melanoma. Ann Surg Oncol. 2016;23(7):2330–5.
27. Kroon HM, Moncrieff M, Kam PCA, Thompson JF. Outcomes following isolated limb infusion for melanoma. A 14-year experience. Ann Surg Oncol. 2008;15(11):3003–13.
28. O'Donoghue C, Perez MC, Mullinax JE, Hardman D, Sileno S, Naqvi SMH, et al. Isolated limb infusion: a single-center experience with over 200 infusions. Ann Surg Oncol. 2017;24(13):3842–9.
29. Miura JT, Kroon HM, Beasley GM, Mullen D, Farrow NE, Mosca PJ, et al. Long-term oncologic outcomes after isolated limb infusion for locoregionally metastatic melanoma: an international multicenter analysis. Ann Surg Oncol. 2019;26(8):2486–94.
30. Ariyan CE, Lefkowitz RA, Panageas K, Callahan MK, Misholy O, Bello D, et al. Safety and clinical activity of combining systemic ipilimumab with isolated limb infusion in patients with in-transit melanoma. J Clin Oncol. 2014;32(15):9078–8.
31. Ariyan CE, Brady MS, Siegelbaum RH, Hu J, Bello DM, Rand J, et al. Robust antitumor responses result from local chemotherapy and CTLA-4 blockade. Cancer Immunol Res. 2018;6(2):189–200.
32. Tan JK, Ho VC. Pooled analysis of the efficacy of bacille Calmette-Guerin (BCG) immunotherapy in malignant melanoma. J Dermatol Surg Oncol. 1993;19(11):985–90.
33. Rosenberg SA, Yang JC, Topalian SL, Schwartzentruber DJ, Weber JS, Parkinson DR, et al. Treatment of 283 consecutive patients with metastatic melanoma or renal cell cancer using high-dose bolus interleukin 2. JAMA. 1994;271(12):907–13.
34. Atkins MB, Lotze MT, Dutcher JP, Fisher RI, Weiss G, Margolin K, et al. High-dose recombinant interleukin 2 therapy for patients with metastatic melanoma: analysis of 270 patients treated between 1985 and 1993. J Clin Oncol. 1999;17(7):2105–16.
35. Davar D, Ding F, Saul M, Sander C, Tarhini AA, Kirkwood JM, et al. High-dose interleukin-2 (HD IL-2) for advanced melanoma: a single center experience from the University of Pittsburgh Cancer Institute. J Immunother Cancer. 2017;5(1):74.
36. Khoury S, Knapp GC, Fyfe A, Monzon J, Temple-Oberle C, McKinnon GJ. Durability of complete response to intralesional interleukin-2 for in-transit melanoma. J Cutan Med Surg. 2021;25(4):364–70.
37. Byers BA, Temple-Oberle CF, Hurdle V, McKinnon JG. Treatment of in-transit melanoma with intra-lesional interleukin-2: a systematic review. J Surg Oncol. 2014;110(6):770–5.

38. Mousavi H, Zhang X, Gillespie S, Wachter E, Hersey P. Rose Bengal induces dual modes of cell death in melanoma cells and has clinical activity against melanoma. Melanoma Res. 2006;16:S8.
39. Thompson JF, Hersey P, Wachter E. Chemoablation of metastatic melanoma using intralesional Rose Bengal. Melanoma Res. 2008;18(6):405–11.
40. Thompson JF, Agarwala SS, Smithers BM, Ross MI, Scoggins CR, Coventry BJ, et al. Phase 2 study of intralesional PV-10 in refractory metastatic melanoma. Ann Surg Oncol. 2015;22(7):2135–42.
41. Dranoff G. GM-CSF-secreting melanoma vaccines. Oncogene. 2003;22(20):3188–92.
42. Grotz TE, Kottschade L, Pavey ES, Markovic SN, Jakub JW. Adjuvant GM-CSF improves survival in high-risk stage IIIC melanoma: a single-center Study. Am J Clin Oncol. 2014;37(5):467–72.
43. Liu BL, Robinson M, Han ZQ, Branston RH, English C, Reay P, et al. ICP34.5 deleted herpes simplex virus with enhanced oncolytic, immune stimulating, and anti-tumour properties. Gene Ther. 2003;10(4):292–303.
44. Harrington KJ, Andtbacka RH, Collichio F, Downey G, Chen L, Szabo Z, et al. Efficacy and safety of talimogene laherparepvec versus granulocyte-macrophage colony-stimulating factor in patients with stage IIIB/C and IVM1a melanoma: subanalysis of the Phase III OPTiM trial. Onco Targets Ther. 2016;9:7081–93.
45. Chesney J, Puzanov I, Collichio F, Singh P, Milhem MM, Glaspy J, et al. Randomized, open-label phase II study evaluating the efficacy and safety of talimogene laherparepvec in combination with ipilimumab versus ipilimumab alone in patients with advanced, unresectable melanoma. J Clin Oncol. 2018;36(17):1658–67.
46. Ribas A, Dummer R, Puzanov I, VanderWalde A, Andtbacka RHI, Michielin O, et al. Oncolytic virotherapy promotes intratumoral T cell infiltration and improves anti-PD-1 Immunotherapy. Cell. 2017;170(6):1109–19.
47. Long GV, Dummer R, Ribas A, Puzanov I, Michielin O, VanderWalde A, et al. A Phase I/III, multicenter, open-label trial of talimogene laherparepvec (T-VEC) in combination with pembrolizumab for the treatment of unresected, stage IIIb-IV melanoma (MASTERKEY-265). J Immunother Cancer. 2015;3(2):181.

Treatment for Stage IV

Introduction

Before the development of small molecule targeted inhibitors and immune checkpoint inhibitors, treatments such as dacarbazine or systemic IL-2 yielded response rates below 20% and led to severe toxicity [1–3]. The discovery of specific gene mutations termed "driver mutations" among several cancers has brought along a more personalized approach to cancer treatment. Likewise, the discovery of the immune checkpoint as a target to increase immune activity against cancer cells has similarly revolutionized treatment of advanced melanoma. Both targeted therapy and immunotherapy achieve substantially improved efficacy and improvement in adverse event profiles compared to previous systemic chemotherapy and systemic IL-2 therapy. Adverse events of systemic targeted and immunotherapy are described in Chap. 7.

Surgery

In some cases, metastatic tumors can be surgically removed, but this is not known to be curative and other treatments are generally required. For decades, complete surgical excision has been the gold standard, even for Stage III or IV cancer [4]. It was typical for positive sentinel lymph node biopsies to be followed by a complete lymph node dissection, a routine based on the observation that patients with macroscopic nodal involvement tended to have worse prognosis [5, 6]. Since then, large, randomized trials have shown no improvement in melanoma-specific survival among patients with melanoma and sentinel-node metastases [7, 8]. Complete lymph node dissection is no longer standard of care for patients with positive SLNB, and adjuvant immunotherapy or targeted therapy is reasonable and effective and spares significant risk of morbidity [9].

Brain Metastases

The brain is a common site of melanoma metastasis and is associated with a poor prognosis with less than 40% of patients surviving at 3 months after a brain metastasis diagnosis [10]. Brain metastases have typically been treated with surgery, whole brain radiotherapy (WBRT), or stereotactic radiosurgery (SRS) [11]. In a study of 115 consecutive melanoma brain metastases patients observed between 1994 and 2010, patients who underwent surgery or SRS had better prognosis than those who received chemotherapy and/or radiotherapy [11]. Common practice is surgical resection for single large brain metastases followed by postoperative SRS given the high rates of recurrence [12, 13]. As an alternative, SRS is recommended for single brain metastases less than 3 cm in diameter with life expectancy greater than 3 months, when metastases are not amenable to surgery, or for 2–4 brain metastases all less than 2.5 cm in diameter in patients with >3-month life expectancy [14]. WBRT can reduce the number of distant metastases and increases local control but does not prolong survival and carries a risk of inducing neurocognitive damage [14].

Targeted Therapy

Targeted treatment agents are administered orally and have a tolerable adverse event profile. A majority of melanomas harbor one of a variety of BRAF mutations. Most clinical trials examining BRAF inhibitors have restricted eligibility to mutations at the BRAF V600 position, which is the most common site [15]. Recent studies have suggested that targeted therapy may also be effective for rarer BRAF mutations [16]. Vemurafenib was approved as the first BRAF inhibitor for treatment of metastatic melanoma in 2011, largely replacing standard chemotherapy as the standard of care for advanced disease in patients harboring the BRAF mutation [17, 18]. Since then, two other BRAF inhibitors have been approved, dabrafenib and encorafenib [19, 20]. The BRAF inhibitors showed great promise because of their high response rates [18–20]. However, it was soon observed that there were high rates of progression, suggesting resistance to BRAF inhibitors [21].

Most cases of BRAF inhibitor resistance are thought to arise from reactivation of the MAPK pathway, increased activation of the PI3K/AKT pathway, or development of other mutations such as in NRAS [22, 23]. Trametinib is an inhibitor of MEK, part of the MAPK pathway, and was shown to improve progression-free survival (PFS) and 6-month overall survival (OS) compared to chemotherapy in patients with BRAF V600 mutations (PFS 4.8 months vs. 1.5 months and OS 81% vs. 67%, respectively) [24]. The combination of BRAF and MEK inhibitors was evaluated in studies with the premise that concurrent MEK inhibition can block reactivation of the MAPK pathway that is upstream of MEK. An open-label study involving 247 patients with metastatic melanoma with BRAF V600 mutations yielded overall response rates (ORR) of 76% for combination treatment compared with 54% for dabrafenib monotherapy [25].

Since then, multiple randomized, phase III trials have shown decreased risk of recurrence in patients with advanced melanoma harboring BRAF V600 mutations. The coBRIM phase III trial showed that the addition of cobimetinib (a MEK inhibitor) to vemurafenib prolongs PFS (12.3 vs. 7.2 months, HR 0.58, 95% CI: 0.46–0.72) and OS (22.3 vs. 17.4 months, HR 0.70, 95% CI 0.55–0.90) compared to vemurafenib monotherapy [26, 27]. Other phase III trials have demonstrated that the combination of dabrafenib and trametinib yields improved OS compared to vemurafenib monotherapy (median OS 25.6 months vs. 18 months) [28, 29]. Similarly, the combination of encorafenib and binimetinib was demonstrated in the COLUMBUS trial to have results consistent with the other BRAF and MEK inhibitor combinations with improved OS and PFS [30]. There are now *three* combinations with FDA approval for unresectable or metastatic melanoma with BRAF V600E or V600K mutations.

Other combinations of targeted therapy have not been able to demonstrate similar consistent results. One nonrandomized multicenter phase II study of trametinib in combination with GSK2141795 (a pan-AKT inhibitor) in patients with NRAS mutant melanoma showed no significant clinical activity [31]. Similar combinations of PI3K inhibitors and MAPK inhibitors have shown mostly disappointing clinical results [32, 33].

Immunotherapy

Melanomas have among the highest rate of mutations of any cancer and produce tumor antigens that are highly immunogenic [34]. Lymphocytes that recognize the diseased cells invade the tissue and are referred to histologically as tumor-infiltrating lymphocytes (TILs). The number of TILs in a tumor is a prognostic indicator for melanoma [35, 36]. T cells require its T-cell receptor to bind an antigen on MHC, along with costimulatory receptor binding to determine its fate. CD28 on the T-cell binding to B7 on an antigen-presenting cell (APC) triggers T-cell activation. Conversely, CTLA-4 on the T cell bound to B7 inhibits T-cell activation.

The first drug in a phase III trial shown to improve overall survival in advanced melanoma was ipilimumab in 2010, a monoclonal antibody targeting CTLA-4 (immune checkpoint inhibitor) [37]. Ipilimumab binds to CTLA-4 and prevents binding with B7, which removes the block on T-cell activation. The median overall survival was 10.1 months for the ipilimumab arm compared to 6.4 months among patients receiving gp100 (a glycoprotein vaccine) in patients who progressed on previous therapy [37]. Ipilimumab has become standard therapy over the past decade for treating metastatic melanoma [38].

Another mechanism of T-cell inhibition is via PD-1 on the T-cell binding to PD-L1 on cells such as cancer cells. One consequence of PD-1 binding to PD-L1 is the prevention of apoptosis of regulatory T cells, which are anti-inflammatory cells that suppress the immune response to host cells [39]. The development of antibodies targeting PD-1 has been hailed as a major advance in cancer therapy, thanks to its impressive efficacy and low toxicity [38]. Two FDA-approved anti-PD-1 antibodies are nivolumab and pembrolizumab. In a large phase I study in which pembrolizumab was evaluated in patients with or without previous ipilimumab treatment, ORR was 40% in the ipilimumab-naïve group and 28% in the ipilimumab-treated group, with a 1-year OS of 71% in all patients [40]. The phase III trial Checkmate-066, which compared nivolumab to dacarbazine chemotherapy in untreated patients with BRAF wild-type melanoma, found an ORR of 40% in the nivolumab group compared with 14% in the dacarbazine group [41]. One-year survival rate was also higher at 73% in the nivolumab group compared with 42% in the dacarbazine group (HR 0.42, $p < 0.001$) [41].

Antibodies to PD-L1 have also been examined in melanoma and results seem promising, but response rates may be lower than those seen with anti-PP-1 antibodies [38]. A phase I study of an anti-PD-L1 antibody in 35 metastatic melanoma patients found an objective response rate of 26%, with some patients demonstrating early tumor shrinkage [42].

Combination Immunotherapy

Combining immune checkpoint inhibitors targeting CTLA-4 and PD-1 was postulated to improve the efficacy in treating metastatic melanoma. The phase III trial Checkmate-067 demonstrated that patients who received the combination of ipilimumab and nivolumab had median OS of more than 60.0 months (median not yet reached at the time of study), compared to 36.9 months (95% CI: 28.2–58.7 months) in the nivolumab group and 19.9 months (95% CI: 16.8–24.6) in the ipilimumab group [43]. An earlier phase I study found that the concurrent combination of the two was shown to have greater objective response rate with tumor reductions of 80% or more and 1-year OS of 94%, compared to 20% in the cohort treated with the combination sequentially [44]. However, the cohort receiving concurrent combination treatment at nivolumab 1 mg/kg and ipilimumab 3 mg/kg experienced relatively high rates of grade 3 or 4 adverse events at 53% [44]. Since then, the Checkmate 511 study has shown decreased incidence of grade 3–5 adverse events with a higher dose of nivolumab (3 mg/kg) and lower dose of ipilimumab (1 mg/kg) without meaningful differences in efficacy [45]. The single-arm Checkmate 204 trial found particular benefit to patients with asymptomatic brain metastases (57% intracranial benefit rate, 26% CR rate) [46, 47]. Based on results of Checkmate-067 and Checkmate-069, the combination of ipilimumab + nivolumab has been recommended for first-line or second-line systemic therapy for unresectable or distant metastatic disease [48].

Several trials are exploring the combination of full dose pembrolizumab (2 mg/kg) with low-dose ipilimumab (1 mg/kg) [48]. The phase IB single-arm open-label trial KEYNOTE-029 showed that for patients with advanced melanoma and no prior checkpoint immunotherapy, the combination of pembrolizumab with ipilimumab resulted in a high response rate, long duration of response (84% of responses lasted at least 36 months), as well as long PFS and OS [49].

Lymphocyte-activating gene 3 (LAG-3) is an inhibitory immune checkpoint like PD-1. The RELATIVITY-047 study is a phase II–III global, double-blind randomized trial that evaluated the combination of nivolumab with a LAG-3 inhibitor relatlimab compared to nivolumab monotherapy and demonstrated increased PFS (10.1 months, 95% CI: 6.4–15.7 vs. 4.6 months, 95% CI: 3.4–5.6) [50]. Findings from this study led to the recent FDA approval of the combination for advanced melanoma.

Combination Targeted and Immunotherapy

Evidence that BRAF inhibitors can improve the efficacy of immunotherapy has led to several studies investigating the combination of targeted therapy and immunotherapy. BRAF mutations may promote immunosuppression via decreased expression of MHC class I [51, 52]. Biopsies of tumors post-BRAF inhibitor treatment were found to have reduced tumor size, enhanced necrosis, and increased T-cell infiltration [52, 53]. BRAF/MEK inhibitor therapy produces a median duration of response between 12 and 18.6 months but, with high rates of developing resistance, may not elicit immunologic memory required for durable antitumor responses [48, 54]. On the other hand, responses to immune checkpoint can take time to develop, with some late responses observed over a year after starting treatment [48].

Combinations of BRAF inhibitor + MEK inhibitor + checkpoint immunotherapy with PD-1 inhibitors (such as pembrolizumab or spartalizumab) or PD-L1 inhibitors (such as atezolizumab) are being studied. Randomized phase II–III trials such as IMspire150, KEYNOTE-022, and COMBI-i have not found improved response rates compared to BRAF/MEK inhibitor doublets, but there was nonsignificant increase PFS without a clear benefit in OS. The KEYNOTE-022 study found nonsignificant increased PFS with the addition of pembrolizumab to dabrafenib plus trametinib compared to the combo of placebo with targeted therapy (16.0 months, 95% CI: 8.6–21.5 months vs. 10.3 months, 95% CI: 7.0–15.6, $p > 0.025$) [55]. The COMBI-i trial investigated the combination of dabrafenib + trametinib with either spartalizumab or placebo but did not find improvement in PFS (HR 0.82, 95% CI: 0.655–1.027, $p > 0.025$) [56]. The IMspire150 randomized double-blind placebo-controlled phase III trial investigated the triplet of vemurafenib + cobimetinib with either atezolizumab or placebo and found significantly improved PFS (15.1 months vs. 10.6 months, HR 0.78, 95% CI: 0.63–0.97, $p = 0.025$) [57]. The IMspire150 study also demonstrated comparable rates of grade 3–4 adverse events between groups (79% in the atezolizumab vs. 73% in the control group) [57]. Based on the IMspire150 study, triplet therapy consisting of atezolizumab plus vemurafenib and cobimetinib has been approved by the FDA and is now among the recommended first-line regimens for BRAF V600 unresectable or metastatic melanoma by NCCN guidelines.

Choosing Therapy

The development of targeted therapy for advanced BRAF V600 mutant melanoma has introduced the idea of personalized therapy for melanoma. Biomarkers such as circulating tumor DNA assays, gene expression profiling, and PD-L1 expression have been studied for guiding therapy [58, 59]. Currently, gene expression profiling and methods of classifying melanoma according to risk of recurrence do not have sufficient evidence for a recommendation in clinical use [60].

The European Society for Medical Oncology (ESMO) in 2019 recommends anti-PD-1 monotherapy or combination anti-PD-1 and anti-CTLA-4 immunotherapy for advanced melanoma with or without BRAF mutations given data demonstrating improved long-term OS [61]. However, patients with rapidly progressive disease or significant contraindications to immunotherapy may be more likely to benefit from combination targeted therapy because of its advantage of having efficacy within the first few months to a year of treatment [61].

A few studies are evaluating options for melanoma disease refractory to immune checkpoint inhibitor therapy. TRIDeNT is a phase II clinical trial exploring the combination of nivolumab plus dabrafenib and trametinib after recurrence or progression on anti-PD-1 therapy [62]. The SECOMBIT phase II trial investigates the various sequences of encorafenib + binimetinib (E+B) and ipilimumab + nivolumab (I+N): arm A with E+B then I+N at progression, arm B with I+N then E+B at progression, and arm C with 8 weeks of E+B, then I+N until progression, and then restarting E+B at progression [63]. With a median follow-up of 37.1 months, early results favor arms B and C for overall survival and time until second progression [63].

References

1. Eggermont AMM, Kirkwood JM. Re-evaluating the role of dacarbazine in metastatic melanoma: what have we learned in 30 years? Eur J Cancer. 2004;40(12):1825–36.
2. Atkins MB, Lotze MT, Dutcher JP, Fisher RI, Weiss G, Margolin K, et al. High-dose recombinant interleukin 2 therapy for patients with metastatic melanoma: analysis of 270 patients treated between 1985 and 1993. J Clin Oncol. 1999;17(7):2105–16.
3. Luikart SD, Kennealey GT, Kirkwood JM. Randomized phase III trial of vinblastine, bleomycin, and cis-dichlorodiammine-platinum versus dacarbazine in malignant melanoma. J Clin Oncol. 1984;2(3):164–8.
4. Testori AAE, Blankenstein SA, van Akkooi ACJ. Surgery for metastatic melanoma: an evolving concept. Curr Oncol Rep. 2019;21(11):98.
5. Morton DL, Thompson JF, Cochran AJ, Mozzillo N, Elashoff R, Essner R, et al. Sentinel-node biopsy or nodal observation in melanoma. N Engl J Med. 2006;355(13):1307–17.
6. Morton DL, Thompson JF, Cochran AJ, Mozzillo N, Nieweg OE, Roses DF, et al. Final trial report of sentinel-node biopsy versus nodal observation in melanoma. N Engl J Med. 2014;370(7):599–609.
7. Faries MB, Thompson JF, Cochran AJ, Andtbacka RH, Mozzillo N, Zager JS, et al. Completion dissection or observation for sentinel-node metastasis in melanoma. N Engl J Med. 2017;376(23):2211–22.

References

8. Leiter U, Stadler R, Mauch C, Hohenberger W, Brockmeyer N, Berking C, et al. Complete lymph node dissection versus no dissection in patients with sentinel lymph node biopsy positive melanoma (DeCOG-SLT): a multicentre, randomised, phase 3 trial. Lancet Oncol. 2016;17(6):757–67.
9. Eggermont AMM, Robert C, Ribas A. The new era of adjuvant therapies for melanoma. Nat Rev Clin Oncol. 2018;15(9):535–6.
10. Ray S, Dacosta-Byfield S, Ganguli A, Bonthapally V, Teitelbaum A. Comparative analysis of survival, treatment, cost and resource use among patients newly diagnosed with brain metastasis by initial primary cancer. J Neuro-Oncol. 2013;114(1):117–25.
11. Vecchio S, Spagnolo F, Merlo DF, Signori A, Acquati M, Pronzato P, et al. The treatment of melanoma brain metastases before the advent of targeted therapies: associations between therapeutic choice, clinical symptoms and outcome with survival. Melanoma Res. 2014;24(1):61–7.
12. Fife K, Colman MH, Stevens GN, Firth IC, Moon D, Shannon KF, et al. Determinants of outcome in melanoma patients with cerebral metastases. J Clin Oncol. 2004;22(7):1293–300.
13. Goldinger SM, Panje C, Nathan P. Treatment of melanoma brain metastases. Curr Opin Oncol. 2016;28(2):159–65.
14. Kocher M, Wittig A, Piroth MD, Treuer H, Seegenschmiedt H, Ruge M, et al. Stereotactic radiosurgery for treatment of brain metastases: a report of the DEGRO Working Group on Stereotactic Radiotherapy. Strahlenther Onkol. 2014;190(6):521–32.
15. Giugliano F, Crimini E, Tarantino P, Zagami P, Uliano J, Corti C, et al. First line treatment of BRAF mutated advanced melanoma: does one size fit all? Cancer Treat Rev. 2021;99:102253.
16. Menzer C, Menzies AM, Carlino MS, Reijers I, Groen EJ, Eigentler T, et al. Targeted therapy in advanced melanoma with rare BRAF mutations. J Clin Oncol. 2019;37(33):3142–51.
17. Chapman PB, Robert C, Larkin J, Haanen JB, Ribas A, Hogg D, et al. Vemurafenib in patients with BRAFV600 mutation-positive metastatic melanoma: final overall survival results of the randomized BRIM-3 study. Ann Oncol. 2017;28(10):2581–7.
18. Chapman PB, Hauschild A, Robert C, Haanen JB, Ascierto P, Larkin J, et al. Improved survival with vemurafenib in melanoma with BRAF V600E mutation. N Engl J Med. 2011;364(26):2507–16.
19. Hauschild A, Grob JJ, Demidov LV, Jouary T, Gutzmer R, Millward M, et al. Dabrafenib in BRAF-mutated metastatic melanoma: a multicentre, open-label, phase 3 randomised controlled trial. Lancet. 2012;380(9839):358–65.
20. Delord JP, Robert C, Nyakas M, McArthur GA, Kudchakar R, Mahipal A, et al. Phase I dose-escalation and -expansion study of the BRAF inhibitor encorafenib (LGX818) in metastatic BRAF-mutant melanoma. Clin Cancer Res. 2017;23(18):5339–48.
21. Fedorenko IV, Paraiso KHT, Smalley KSM. Acquired and intrinsic BRAF inhibitor resistance in BRAF V600E mutant melanoma. Biochem Pharmacol. 2011;82(3):201–9.
22. Chapman PB. Mechanisms of resistance to RAF inhibition in melanomas harboring a BRAF mutation. Am Soc Clin Oncol Educ Book. 2013. https://doi.org/10.1200/EdBook_AM.2013.33.e80.
23. Atefi M, von Euw E, Attar N, Ng C, Chu C, Guo D, et al. Reversing melanoma cross-resistance to BRAF and MEK inhibitors by co-targeting the AKT/mTOR pathway. PLoS One. 2011;6(12):e28973.
24. Flaherty KT, Robert C, Hersey P, Nathan P, Garbe C, Milhem M, et al. Improved survival with MEK inhibition in BRAF-mutated melanoma. N Engl J Med. 2012;367(2):107–14.
25. Flaherty KT, Infante JR, Daud A, Gonzalez R, Kefford RF, Sosman J, et al. Combined BRAF and MEK inhibition in melanoma with BRAF V600 mutations. N Engl J Med. 2012;367(18):1694–703.
26. Ascierto PA, McArthur GA, Dréno B, Atkinson V, Liszkay G, Di Giacomo AM, et al. Cobimetinib combined with vemurafenib in advanced BRAF(V600)-mutant melanoma (coBRIM): updated efficacy results from a randomised, double-blind, phase 3 trial. Lancet Oncol. 2016;17(9):1248–60.
27. Larkin J, Ascierto PA, Dréno B, Atkinson V, Liszkay G, Maio M, et al. Combined vemurafenib and cobimetinib in BRAF-mutated melanoma. N Engl J Med. 2014;371(20):1867–76.

28. Long GV, Hauschild A, Santinami M, Atkinson V, Mandalà M, Chiarion-Sileni V, et al. Adjuvant dabrafenib plus trametinib in stage III BRAF-mutated melanoma. N Engl J Med. 2017;377(19):1813–23.
29. Robert C, Karaszewska B, Schachter J, Rutkowski P, Mackiewicz A, Stroiakovski D, et al. Improved overall survival in melanoma with combined dabrafenib and trametinib. N Engl J Med. 2015;372(1):30–9.
30. Ascierto PA, Dummer R, Gogas HJ, Flaherty KT, Arance A, Mandala M, et al. Update on tolerability and overall survival in COLUMBUS: landmark analysis of a randomised phase 3 trial of encorafenib plus binimetinib vs vemurafenib or encorafenib in patients with BRAF V600-mutant melanoma. Eur J Cancer. 1990;2020(126):33–44.
31. Algazi AP, Esteve-Puig R, Nosrati A, Hinds B, Hobbs-Muthukumar A, Nandoskar P, et al. Dual MEK/AKT inhibition with trametinib and GSK2141795 does not yield clinical benefit in metastatic NRAS-mutant and wild-type melanoma. Pigment Cell Melanoma Res. 2018;31(1):110–4.
32. Lim SY, Menzies AM, Rizos H. Mechanisms and strategies to overcome resistance to molecularly targeted therapy for melanoma. Cancer. 2017;123(S11):2118–29.
33. Tolcher AW, Patnaik A, Papadopoulos KP, Rasco DW, Becerra CR, Allred AJ, et al. Phase I study of the MEK inhibitor trametinib in combination with the AKT inhibitor afuresertib in patients with solid tumors and multiple myeloma. Cancer Chemother Pharmacol. 2015;75(1):183–9.
34. Alexandrov LB, Nik-Zainal S, Wedge DC, Aparicio SAJR, Behjati S, Biankin AV, et al. Signatures of mutational processes in human cancer. Nature. 2013;500(7463):415–21.
35. Lee N, Zakka LR, Mihm MC, Schatton T. Tumour-infiltrating lymphocytes in melanoma prognosis and cancer immunotherapy. Pathology. 2016;48(2):177–87.
36. Fu Q, Chen N, Ge C, Li R, Li Z, Zeng B, et al. Prognostic value of tumor-infiltrating lymphocytes in melanoma: a systematic review and meta-analysis. Onco Targets Ther. 2019;8(7):1593806.
37. Hodi FS, O'Day SJ, McDermott DF, Weber RW, Sosman JA, Haanen JB, et al. Improved survival with ipilimumab in patients with metastatic melanoma. N Engl J Med. 2010;363(8):711–23.
38. Carlino MS, Larkin J, Long GV. Immune checkpoint inhibitors in melanoma. Lancet. 2021;398(10304):1002–14.
39. Passarelli A, Mannavola F, Stucci LS, Tucci M, Silvestris F. Immune system and melanoma biology: a balance between immunosurveillance and immune escape. Oncotarget. 2017;8(62):106132–42.
40. Ribas A, Hodi FS, Kefford R, Hamid O, Daud A, Wolchok JD, et al. Efficacy and safety of the anti-PD-1 monoclonal antibody MK-3475 in 411 patients (pts) with melanoma (MEL). J Clin Oncol. 2014;32(18):LBA9000.
41. Robert C, Long GV, Brady B, Dutriaux C, Maio M, Mortier L, et al. Nivolumab in previously untreated melanoma without BRAF mutation. N Engl J Med. 2015;372(4):320–30.
42. Hamid O, Sosman J, Lawrence D, Sullivan R, Ibrahim N, Kluger H, et al. Clinical activity, safety, and biomarkers of MPDL3280A, an engineered PD-L1 antibody in patients with locally advanced or metastatic melanoma (mM). J Clin Oncol. 2013;31(15):9010.
43. Larkin J, Chiarion-Sileni V, Gonzalez R, Grob JJ, Rutkowski P, Lao CD, et al. Five-year survival with combined nivolumab and ipilimumab in advanced melanoma. N Engl J Med. 2019;381(16):1535–46.
44. Wolchok JD, Kluger H, Callahan MK, Postow MA, Rizvi NA, Lesokhin AM, et al. Nivolumab plus ipilimumab in advanced melanoma. N Engl J Med. 2013;369(2):122–33.
45. Lebbé C, Meyer N, Mortier L, Marquez-Rodas I, Robert C, Rutkowski P, et al. Evaluation of two dosing regimens for nivolumab in combination with ipilimumab in patients with advanced melanoma: results from the phase IIIb/IV CheckMate 511 trial. J Clin Oncol. 2019;37(11):867–75.
46. Tawbi HA, Forsyth PA, Algazi A, Hamid O, Hodi FS, Moschos SJ, et al. Combined nivolumab and ipilimumab in melanoma metastatic to the brain. N Engl J Med. 2018;379(8):722–30.
47. Tawbi HA, Forsyth PA, Hodi FS, Algazi AP, Hamid O, Lao CD, et al. Long-term outcomes of patients with active melanoma brain metastases treated with combination nivolumab plus

ipilimumab (CheckMate 204): final results of an open-label, multicentre, phase 2 study. Lancet Oncol. 2021;22(12):1692–704.
48. Swetter SM, Thompson JA, Albertini MR, Barker CA, Baumgartner J, Boland G, et al. NCCN guidelines® insights: melanoma: cutaneous, version 2.2021: featured updates to the NCCN guidelines. J Natl Compr Cancer Netw. 2021;19(4):364–76.
49. Long GV, Atkinson V, Cebon JS, Jameson MB, Fitzharris BM, McNeil CM, et al. Standard-dose pembrolizumab in combination with reduced-dose ipilimumab for patients with advanced melanoma (KEYNOTE-029): an open-label, phase 1b trial. Lancet Oncol. 2017;18(9):1202–10.
50. Tawbi HA, Schadendorf D, Lipson EJ, Ascierto PA, Matamala L, Castillo Gutiérrez E, et al. Relatlimab and nivolumab versus nivolumab in untreated advanced melanoma. N Engl J Med. 2022;386(1):24–34.
51. Bradley SD, Chen Z, Melendez B, Talukder A, Khalili JS, Rodriguez-Cruz T, et al. BRAFV600E Co-opts a conserved MHC class I internalization pathway to diminish antigen presentation and CD8+ T-cell recognition of melanoma. Cancer Immunol Res. 2015;3(6):602–9.
52. Wilmott JS, Long GV, Howle JR, Haydu LE, Sharma RN, Thompson JF, et al. Selective BRAF inhibitors induce marked T-cell infiltration into human metastatic melanoma. Clin Cancer Res. 2012;18(5):1386–94.
53. Liu C, Peng W, Xu C, Lou Y, Zhang M, Wargo JA, et al. BRAF inhibition increases tumor infiltration by T cells and enhances the antitumor activity of adoptive immunotherapy in mice. Clin Cancer Res. 2013;19(2):393–403.
54. Long GV, Stroyakovskiy D, Gogas H, Levchenko E, de Braud F, Larkin J, et al. Dabrafenib and trametinib versus dabrafenib and placebo for Val600 BRAF-mutant melanoma: a multicentre, double-blind, phase 3 randomised controlled trial. Lancet. 2015;386(9992):444–51.
55. Ferrucci PF, Di Giacomo AM, Del Vecchio M, Atkinson V, Schmidt H, Schachter J, et al. KEYNOTE-022 part 3: a randomized, double-blind, phase 2 study of pembrolizumab, dabrafenib, and trametinib in BRAF-mutant melanoma. J Immunother Cancer. 2020;8(2):e001806.
56. Nathan P, Dummer R, Long GV, Ascierto PA, Tawbi HA, Robert C, et al. LBA43 Spartalizumab plus dabrafenib and trametinib (Sparta-DabTram) in patients (pts) with previously untreated BRAF V600–mutant unresectable or metastatic melanoma: results from the randomized part 3 of the phase III COMBI-I trial. Ann Oncol. 2020;31:S1172.
57. Gutzmer R, Stroyakovskiy D, Gogas H, Robert C, Lewis K, Protsenko S, et al. Atezolizumab, vemurafenib, and cobimetinib as first-line treatment for unresectable advanced BRAFV600 mutation-positive melanoma (IMspire150): primary analysis of the randomised, double-blind, placebo-controlled, phase 3 trial. Lancet. 2020;395(10240):1835–44.
58. Gibney GT, Weiner LM, Atkins MB. Predictive biomarkers for checkpoint inhibitor-based immunotherapy. Lancet Oncol. 2016;17(12):e542–51.
59. Paver EC, Cooper WA, Colebatch AJ, Ferguson PM, Hill SK, Lum T, et al. Programmed death ligand-1 (PD-L1) as a predictive marker for immunotherapy in solid tumours: a guide to immunohistochemistry implementation and interpretation. Pathology. 2021;53(2):141–56.
60. Grossman D, Okwundu N, Bartlett EK, Marchetti MA, Othus M, Coit DG, et al. Prognostic gene expression profiling in cutaneous melanoma: identifying the knowledge gaps and assessing the clinical benefit. JAMA Dermatol. 2020;156(9):1004.
61. Michielin O, van Akkooi ACJ, Ascierto PA, Dummer R, Keilholz U, ESMO Guidelines Committee. Cutaneous melanoma: ESMO clinical practice guidelines for diagnosis, treatment and follow-up. Ann Oncol. 2019;30(12):1884–901.
62. Burton EM, Amaria RN, Glitza IC, Milton DR, Diab A, Patel SP, et al. Phase II study of TRIplet combination Nivolumab (N) with Dabrafenib (D) and Trametinib (T) (TRIDeNT) in patients (pts) with PD-1 naïve or refractory BRAF-mutated metastatic melanoma (MM) with or without active brain metastases. J Clin Oncol. 2021;39(15):9520.
63. Ascierto PA, Mandalà M, Ferrucci PF, Guidoboni M, Rutkowski P, Ferraresi V, et al. Phase II study SECOMBIT (sequential combo immuno and target therapy study): a subgroup analysis with a longer follow-up. J Clin Oncol. 2022;40:9535. https://ascopubs.org/doi/pdf/10.1200/JCO.2022.40.16_suppl.9535.

Side Effects of Melanoma Therapy

Targeted Therapy

The use of BRAF inhibitors was previously found to be associated with the development of cutaneous squamous cell carcinoma and keratoacanthoma, likely due to rapid reactivation of the MAPK pathway in BRAF wild-type cells [1, 2]. This was more common with vemurafenib (20%) than dabrafenib (6%) or encorafenib (3%) [3–5]. Combining MEK inhibitors with BRAF inhibitors decreased rates of SCC and keratoacanthoma compared to BRAF inhibitor monotherapy, but was associated with higher rates of pyrexia, photosensitivity, and gastrointestinal toxicities [6–8].

The phase III coBRIM trial found that the common adverse events associated with the combination of vemurafenib and cobimetinib included rash (73%), diarrhea (61%), photosensitivity (34%), elevated creatine phosphokinase, serous retinopathy, pyrexia, and elevated alanine aminotransferase (ALT) [9, 10]. Adverse events most commonly present in the first 28 days of treatment and decrease substantially over time [9]. Treatment for the adverse events from the coBRIM trial included supportive care, dose modifications, or treatment discontinuation [9]. Elevated liver enzymes were managed with vemurafenib dose modification. Elevated creatine kinase was managed by interrupting or reducing cobimetinib and uncommonly discontinuation. Photosensitivity was managed conservatively with few patients requiring dose modification. Serous retinopathy was managed by close observation and cobimetinib dose modification. One case of retinal ischemia did not need treatment modification and resolved while continuing treatment. Reduced left ventricular was managed by cobimetinib dose modification or discontinuation. Diarrhea was managed with loperamide. Squamous cell carcinoma and keratoacanthoma were treated surgically with complete excision. With the sole exception of rash, most patients did not have recurrence of adverse events after dose modification or conservative management [9].

Immune Checkpoint Inhibitors

By reducing T-cell suppression, immune checkpoint inhibitors increase the potential for inflammatory damage to various organs. Dermatologic toxicities were most common with up to 50% of treated patients experiencing rash, pruritus, dermatitis, vitiligo, or bullous dermatitis [11]. However, it should be noted that vitiligo is associated with improved prognosis and predicts regression of tumor and prolonged survival [12]. The colon is the next most commonly affected organ and up to 40% of patients receiving immune checkpoint inhibitor therapy may develop colitis, which presents as diarrhea [13]. Hepatitis and pancreatitis may occur presenting as transaminitis or elevated amylase and lipase, respectively [14]. Pulmonary adverse events include pneumonitis and sarcoidosis [15, 16]. Rheumatologic and musculoskeletal adverse events may also occur and include oligo- or polyarthritis, a polymyalgia rheumatica-type syndrome, sicca syndrome, and inflammatory myositis with fasciitis [17]. Renal injury presents as acute kidney injury, with AKI Stage I rates of 24.5–29% and AKI Stage II rates of 5–10% [18].

Rarer adverse events (<1%) included immunologic effects ophthalmologically, neurologically, cardiac, and hematologic. Ophthalmic adverse events include vision alteration, optic nerve swelling, uveitis, episcleritis, and blepharitis [19]. Neurologic adverse events are also rare and include myasthenia gravis, Guillain-Barre syndrome, encephalitis, aseptic meningitis, hypophysitis, and transverse myelitis [20]. Cardiac adverse events include heart failure, cardiomyopathy, heart block, myocardial fibrosis, and myocarditis [21]. Hematologic adverse events include neutropenia, autoimmune hemolytic anemia, immune thrombocytopenia, and aplastic anemia [22].

The adverse events for CTLA-4 inhibitors such as ipilimumab were found to be colitis, dermatitis, hepatitis, hypophysitis, thyroiditis, and adrenal insufficiency [23]. Phase III trials show that grade 3 or 4 immune-related adverse events occurred in 10–15% of patients in ipilimumab group [24, 25]. The Keynote 006 trial found that the most frequent adverse events for patients on ipilimumab were pruritus (25.4%), diarrhea (22.7%), fatigue (15.2%), and rash (14.5) [26]. Monitoring patients for colitis and treating with corticosteroids may prevent progression to bowel perforation and death [23, 27]. While colitis, dermatitis, and hepatitis are generally reversible with steroids, side effects such as hypophysitis or hypothyroidism may require lifelong hormone replacement therapy [23]. Previous attempts at combining a CTLA-4 inhibitor with a BRAF inhibitor have required early termination of the trial because of high rates of hepatotoxicity [28].

PD-1 inhibitors are considered to have lower toxicity than CTLA-4 inhibitors. The Checkmate-511 trial showed that a higher dose of nivolumab with a lower dose of ipilimumab significantly reduced the rate of adverse events compared to a higher dose of ipilimumab and lower dose of nivolumab [29]. The Keynote 006 trial showed that pembrolizumab was associated with lower rates of permanent discontinuation than ipilimumab (4.0–6.9% for pembrolizumab vs. 9.4% for ipilimumab) [26]. The most common treatment-related adverse events for patients on pembrolizumab include fatigue (19.1–20.9%), diarrhea (14.4–16.9%), rash (13.4–14.7%), and pruritis (14.1–14.4%) [26]. This reflected a previous phase I/II study of 107 patients showed that the most common adverse events with nivolumab were fatigue, rash, and diarrhea [30]. One of the most concerning potential toxicities with PD-1 inhibitors is pneumonitis, as a phase I trial of nivolumab in several cancer types found 3% of patients developing pneumonitis, including 3 of 296 patients (2 of whom had lung cancer, none with melanoma) developing fatal pulmonary toxicity [31]. Low-grade pneumonitis was successfully managed by interruption of treatment and/or corticosteroid treatment.

References

1. Adelmann CH, Ching G, Du L, Saporito RC, Bansal V, Pence LJ, et al. Comparative profiles of BRAF inhibitors: the paradox index as a predictor of clinical toxicity. Oncotarget. 2016;7(21):30453–60.
2. Su F, Viros A, Milagre C, Trunzer K, Bollag G, Spleiss O, et al. RAS mutations in cutaneous squamous-cell carcinomas in patients treated with BRAF inhibitors. N Engl J Med. 2012;366(3):207–15.
3. Chapman PB, Hauschild A, Robert C, Haanen JB, Ascierto P, Larkin J, et al. Improved survival with vemurafenib in melanoma with BRAF V600E mutation. N Engl J Med. 2011;364(26):2507–16.
4. Hauschild A, Grob JJ, Demidov LV, Jouary T, Gutzmer R, Millward M, et al. Dabrafenib in BRAF-mutated metastatic melanoma: a multicentre, open-label, phase 3 randomised controlled trial. Lancet Lond Engl. 2012;380(9839):358–65.
5. Delord JP, Robert C, Nyakas M, McArthur GA, Kudchakar R, Mahipal A, et al. Phase I dose-escalation and -expansion study of the BRAF inhibitor Encorafenib (LGX818) in metastatic BRAF-mutant melanoma. Clin Cancer Res. 2017;23(18):5339–48.
6. Ascierto PA, McArthur GA, Dréno B, Atkinson V, Liszkay G, Di Giacomo AM, et al. Cobimetinib combined with vemurafenib in advanced BRAF(V600)-mutant melanoma (coBRIM): updated efficacy results from a randomised, double-blind, phase 3 trial. Lancet Oncol. 2016;17(9):1248–60.
7. Robert C, Grob JJ, Stroyakovskiy D, Karaszewska B, Hauschild A, Levchenko E, et al. Five-year outcomes with Dabrafenib plus Trametinib in metastatic melanoma. N Engl J Med. 2019;381(7):626–36.
8. Ascierto PA, Dummer R. Immunological effects of BRAF+MEK inhibition. Onco Targets Ther. 2018;7(9):e1468955.
9. Dréno B, Ribas A, Larkin J, Ascierto PA, Hauschild A, Thomas L, et al. Incidence, course, and management of toxicities associated with cobimetinib in combination with vemurafenib in the coBRIM study. Ann Oncol. 2017;28(5):1137–44.
10. Giugliano F, Crimini E, Tarantino P, Zagami P, Uliano J, Corti C, et al. First line treatment of BRAF mutated advanced melanoma: does one size fit all? Cancer Treat Rev. 2021;99:102253.
11. Ralli M, Botticelli A, Visconti IC, Angeletti D, Fiore M, Marchetti P, et al. Immunotherapy in the treatment of metastatic melanoma: current knowledge and future directions. J Immunol Res. 2020;2020:1–12.
12. Teulings HE, Limpens J, Jansen SN, Zwinderman AH, Reitsma JB, Spuls PI, et al. Vitiligo-like depigmentation in patients with stage III-IV melanoma receiving immunotherapy and its association with survival: a systematic review and meta-analysis. J Clin Oncol. 2015;33(7):773–81.
13. Shivaji UN, Jeffery L, Gui X, Smith SCL, Ahmad OF, Akbar A, et al. Immune checkpoint inhibitor-associated gastrointestinal and hepatic adverse events and their management. Ther Adv Gastroenterol. 2019;12:1756284819884196.

14. Rajha E, Chaftari P, Kamal M, Maamari J, Chaftari C, Yeung SCJ. Gastrointestinal adverse events associated with immune checkpoint inhibitor therapy. Gastroenterol Rep. 2020;8(1):25–30.
15. Jain A, Shannon VR, Sheshadri A. Immune-related adverse events: pneumonitis. Adv Exp Med Biol. 2018;995:131–49.
16. Rashdan S, Minna JD, Gerber DE. Diagnosis and management of pulmonary toxicity associated with cancer immunotherapy. Lancet Respir Med. 2018;6(6):472–8.
17. Narváez J, Juarez-López P, LLuch J, Narváez JA, Palmero R, García Del Muro X, et al. Rheumatic immune-related adverse events in patients on anti-PD-1 inhibitors: fasciitis with myositis syndrome as a new complication of immunotherapy. Autoimmun Rev. 2018;17(10):1040–5.
18. Wanchoo R, Karam S, Uppal NN, Barta VS, Deray G, Devoe C, et al. Adverse renal effects of immune checkpoint inhibitors: a narrative review. Am J Nephrol. 2017;45(2):160–9.
19. Fang T, Maberley DA, Etminan M. Ocular adverse events with immune checkpoint inhibitors. J Curr Ophthalmol. 2019;31(3):319–22.
20. Pan PCW, Haggiagi A. Neurologic immune-related adverse events associated with immune checkpoint inhibition. Curr Oncol Rep. 2019;21(12):108.
21. Heinzerling L, Ott PA, Hodi FS, Husain AN, Tajmir-Riahi A, Tawbi H, et al. Cardiotoxicity associated with CTLA4 and PD1 blocking immunotherapy. J Immunother Cancer. 2016;4:50.
22. Delanoy N, Michot JM, Comont T, Kramkimel N, Lazarovici J, Dupont R, et al. Haematological immune-related adverse events induced by anti-PD-1 or anti-PD-L1 immunotherapy: a descriptive observational study. Lancet Haematol. 2019;6(1):e48–57.
23. Carlino MS, Larkin J, Long GV. Immune checkpoint inhibitors in melanoma. Lancet. 2021;398(10304):1002–14.
24. Hodi FS, O'Day SJ, McDermott DF, Weber RW, Sosman JA, Haanen JB, et al. Improved survival with ipilimumab in patients with metastatic melanoma. N Engl J Med. 2010;363(8):711–23.
25. Robert C, Thomas L, Bondarenko I, O'Day S, Weber J, Garbe C, et al. Ipilimumab plus dacarbazine for previously untreated metastatic melanoma. N Engl J Med. 2011;364(26):2517–26.
26. Robert C, Schachter J, Long GV, Arance A, Grob JJ, Mortier L, et al. Pembrolizumab versus ipilimumab in advanced melanoma. N Engl J Med. 2015;372(26):2521–32.
27. Weber JS, Kähler KC, Hauschild A. Management of immune-related adverse events and kinetics of response with ipilimumab. J Clin Oncol Off J Am Soc Clin Oncol. 2012;30(21):2691–7.
28. Ribas A, Hodi FS, Callahan M, Konto C, Wolchok J. Hepatotoxicity with combination of vemurafenib and ipilimumab. N Engl J Med. 2013;368(14):1365–6.
29. Swetter SM, Thompson JA, Albertini MR, Barker CA, Baumgartner J, Boland G, et al. NCCN guidelines® insights: melanoma: cutaneous, version 2.2021: featured updates to the NCCN guidelines. J Natl Compr Cancer Netw. 2021;19(4):364–76.
30. Topalian SL, Sznol M, McDermott DF, Kluger HM, Carvajal RD, Sharfman WH, et al. Survival, durable tumor remission, and long-term safety in patients with advanced melanoma receiving nivolumab. J Clin Oncol Off J Am Soc Clin Oncol. 2014;32(10):1020–30.
31. Hamid O, Sosman J, Lawrence D, Sullivan R, Ibrahim N, Kluger H, et al. Clinical activity, safety, and biomarkers of MPDL3280A, an engineered PD-L1 antibody in patients with locally advanced or metastatic melanoma (mM). J Clin Oncol. 2013;31(15Suppl):9010.

Pediatric Melanoma

8

Pediatric melanoma is thought to be a rare childhood neoplasm with a mere 1317 cases recorded between 1973 and 2009 in the Surveillance, Epidemiology, and End Results (SEER) Program data [1]. Annual incidence is estimated to be approximately 1–3% of total pediatric malignancies, with a large majority consisting of postpubescent cases [2–7]. While rare, pediatric melanoma has been increasing in incidence by an average of 2% per year and clinicians must continue to remain vigilant for melanoma in the pediatric population [2, 4].

In addition to its relative rarity, pediatric melanoma's variance in presentation, survival rates, and risk factors versus that of adult cases hinders its detection. While not all physicians will be confronted with this malignancy, it is crucial that they understand the population-specific considerations to ensure timely detection and treatment.

Clinical Presentation

Pediatric melanoma has less clear-cut clinical features and more variance in presentation. Unlike adult melanoma that typically conforms to the conventional ABCDE (*A*symmetry, *B*order, *C*olor, *D*iameter, *E*volving) mnemonic of melanoma [8–10], pediatric melanoma does not always conform and can present with unconventional features like amelanosis, ulceration, bumps, uniformity in color, variable diameter, and de novo development [11]. According to a large retrospective study of children with melanoma, 60% of cases aged 10 years and under lacked ABCDE criteria and 77% were amelanotic compared to 40% and 23% of cases between 11 and 19 years of age [11]. The presence of unconventional features means pediatric melanoma can appear similar to other nonmelanocytic lesions including angiomas, pyogenic granulomas, viral warts, and some Spitz nevi [12–14]. Additional ABCD (*A*melanotic, *B*leeding or *B*ump, *C*olor uniformity, *D*e novo, any *D*iameter) detection criteria have been proposed to raise awareness of the alternate presentations of melanoma in children [11].

Of the clinically similar lesions, Spitz nevi are particularly problematic. Originally coined "Spitz lesion" to refer to "melanomas of childhood," Spitz nevi are now classified as benign melanocytic nevi that occur in children and adults [15, 16]. They typically present as solitary, pink-red or brown lesions on the lower extremities, trunk, and head and neck region (particularly for children) [16–19]. While Spitz nevi themselves are not problematic, there exists a spectrum of Spitz-type lesions ranging from benign Spitz nevi to Spitzoid melanoma, with atypical Spitz tumor (AST) or melanocytic tumors of uncertain malignant potential (MELTUMPs) occupying the middle of the spectrum [20]. Lesions on this spectrum can be difficult to distinguish, with no distinct immunohistochemical or molecular markers and poorly predictive histopathologic and dermatoscopic features for ambiguous lesions [17, 18, 20, 21]. Management of Spitz nevi is age dependent as children are much more likely to develop Spitz nevi, while adults are much more likely to develop melanoma [19–22]. Wide local excision is recommended for adults with Spitz nevi and can be considered for atypical lesions in children over 12 years of age [23–25]. For the pediatric population, regular dermatoscopic examination (for children younger than 12 years of age) and partial biopsy have been proposed as alternatives to total biopsy by some experts [24, 26, 27]. However, Spitz nevi with atypical characteristics including those that are larger, nodular, changing, bleeding, and ulcerated or have other concerning features should be biopsied with margins [28]. Sentinel lymph node biopsy has uncertain survival benefit and should be considered on a case-by-case basis [21, 29].

Congenital melanocytic nevi (CMN) are another lesion of special interest within the pediatric population. CMN are pigmented lesions that are present at birth or appear within the first year of life and are classified as small (<1.5 cm), medium (1.5–20 cm), large (>20 cm), and giant (>40–60 cm) based on projected adult size. They occur in 1 in 20,000 to 1 in 500,000 newborns [30]. Common features include size larger than common nevi, color variegation, hypertrichosis, and "cobblestone pattern" by dermoscopy [31]. The risk of developing melanoma correlates with CMN size. Literature suggests that pediatric patients with small and medium CMN have a fairly low risk of developing melanoma, while patients with large CMN are at a significantly higher risk of developing melanoma with a risk maximum in childhood and adolescence [28, 30, 32–34]. Additionally, there is evidence that melanomas tend to arise at younger ages in patients with large CMN and primarily after puberty for patients with smaller CMN [31]. Given the behavior of CMN, treatment should be determined case-by-case by weighing melanoma risk against aesthetic and psychosocial considerations. For smaller CMN, regular follow-up is sufficient for management though excision may also be considered [30, 31]. For large CMN, excision can be considered as prophylaxis against subsequent transformation into melanoma; however, patients and parents should be counseled that excision cannot completely ameliorate the risk of transformation [30, 31].

Risk Factors

Risk factors for pediatric melanoma remain generally the same as those of adult melanoma (further discussed in Chap. 16) and include non-modifiable (age, family history, pigmentation, nevi pattern) and modifiable (sun exposure and phototoxic medications) factors. Despite the similarities, clinicals must be aware of pediatric specific trends in risk, which may suggest potential biological differences between pediatric and adult melanoma.

While the risk of melanoma is generally low in children, the risk increases with age and shows a clear cutoff represented by puberty [31, 35]. Familial history has been demonstrated to be an important risk factor for children of all ages in multiple studies; however, inactivation of the CDKN2A gene, typically associated with hereditary melanoma, was only present in 5% of pediatric cases observed in one study suggesting different genetic underpinnings for early-onset melanoma [3, 11, 36]. Children, just as adults, with Fitzpatrick I (fair skin with blonde or red hair), followed by those who burn easily, tan poorly, and freckle are at the highest risk of developing melanoma [11, 37]. It is important to note that darker-skinned children are still at risk of developing melanoma, with the highest incidence observed in the youngest age groups of one study and a subsequent decline observed with increasing age [11]. This unusual finding again suggests potential differences in biological underpinnings. Additionally, history of greater than 3 sunburns and increased UV exposure are also associated with increased risk of melanoma, particularly in older, adolescent children [3, 5, 11]. This bias suggests a larger influence of environmental exposure for older children while suggesting a larger genetic role in younger children [11]. Due to this association, patients at higher risk should be counseled to avoid sunburns, phototoxic medications, and other UV exposure like tanning bed use [28, 38]. Other risk factors include high number of acquired melanocytic nevi or dysplastic nevi and presence of CMN, particularly large ones [11, 30].

Prognosis

Reports on the prognosis for melanoma in children vary within current literature, generally reporting same if not better behavior versus that of adult populations. Despite observing thicker primary lesions, more frequent nodal metastasis, and histologically aggressive features (ulceration, mitosis) in younger children, multiple studies observe higher survival in younger patients (typically at or under 10 years of age) [11, 12, 14, 39, 40]. These differences could suggest biological differences between melanoma of young children and those of adolescents and adults, though further data is required to support this hypothesis [12, 41]. Other studies observe similar prognosis between pediatric and adult melanoma cases [28, 42–44]. Part, though not all, of this difference may be attributed to the higher prevalence of ambiguous lesions and melanoma mimics resulting in a tendency to overdiagnose

[45] and a need to excise 20-times more lesions to detect one melanoma in pediatric populations [46]. Further complicating prognosis is the differing behavior observed among different histological subtypes of pediatric melanoma with worse survival noted for nodular and congenital nevus-associated melanoma [47]. Further research into prognosis is crucial as utilizing adult-based protocols for treating pediatric melanoma may lead to overtreatment and unnecessary morbidity if melanoma does indeed have a better prognosis within children [41].

Management

Because of the rarity of melanoma within the pediatric population, screening is not routinely recommended before puberty. For children at an elevated risk for melanoma, definitive guidelines do not currently exist for screening [48]. A combination of home self-monitoring and subsequent dermatologic evaluation of suspicious lesions has been proposed within literature [28, 48]. Once puberty is reached, routine clinical follow-up is recommended for high-risk adolescents [31]. Patients, caregivers, and providers should be aware of the differing behavior of pediatric melanoma discussed earlier when evaluating lesions, including the expanded ABCD proposed by Cordoro et al. [11]. Atypical Spitz nevi should be biopsied until their malignant potential can be better characterized. Patients with large CMN should have annual clinical follow-up due to both increased risk and poorer prognosis discussed earlier. Overall, it is recommended that any thick, ulcerated, nodular lesions should be excised at any age [31]. For other lesions, a combination of history, clinical and dermatoscopic features, aesthetic, and psychosocial factors should be considered before excising a lesion.

Treatment of pediatric melanoma utilizes similar modalities to that of adult melanomas though importance of sentinel lymph node biopsy (SLNB) and use of adjuvant therapies requires further clarification due to differing reports on the significance of positive lymph nodes as a prognostic factor for pediatric melanoma [5, 42, 49, 50].

References

1. Wong JR, Harris JK, Rodriguez-Galindo C, Johnson KJ. Incidence of childhood and adolescent melanoma in the United States: 1973–2009. Pediatrics. 2013;131(5):846–54.
2. Rao BN, Hayes FA, Pratt CB, Fleming ID, Kumar APM, Lobe T, et al. Malignant melanoma in children: Its management and prognosis. J Pediatr Surg. 1990;25(2):198–203.
3. Pappo AS. Melanoma in children and adolescents. Eur J Cancer. 2003;39(18):2651–61.
4. Lange JR, Balch CM. Melanoma in children: heightened awareness of an uncommon but often curable malignancy. Pediatrics. 2005;115(3):802–3.
5. Strouse JJ, Fears TR, Tucker MA, Wayne AS. Pediatric melanoma: risk factor and survival analysis of the surveillance, epidemiology and end results database. J Clin Oncol. 2005;23(21):4735–41.
6. Huynh PM, Grant-Kels JM, Grin CM. Childhood melanoma: update and treatment. Int J Dermatol. 2005;44(9):715–23.

References

7. Schaffer JV. Pigmented lesions in children: when to worry. Curr Opin Pediatr. 2007;19(4):430–40.
8. Friedman RJ, Rigel DS, Kopf AW. Early detection of malignant melanoma: the role of physician examination and self-examination of the skin. CA Cancer J Clin. 1985;35(3):130–51.
9. Abbasi NR, Shaw HM, Rigel DS, Friedman RJ, McCarthy WH, Osman I, et al. Early diagnosis of cutaneous melanoma revisiting the ABCD criteria. JAMA. 2004;292(22):2771–6.
10. Tsao H, Olazagasti JM, Cordoro KM, Brewer JD, Taylor SC, Bordeaux JS, et al. Early detection of melanoma: reviewing the ABCDEs. J Am Acad Dermatol. 2015;72(4):717–23.
11. Cordoro KM, Gupta D, Frieden IJ, McCalmont T, Kashani-Sabet M. Pediatric melanoma: results of a large cohort study and proposal for modified ABCD detection criteria for children. J Am Acad Dermatol. 2013;68(6):913–25.
12. Ferrari A, Bono A, Baldi M, Collini P, Casanova M, Pennacchioli E, et al. Does melanoma behave differently in younger children than in adults? A retrospective study of 33 cases of childhood melanoma from a single institution. Pediatrics. 2005;115(3):649–54.
13. Mones JM, Ackerman AB. Melanomas in prepubescent children: review comprehensively, critique historically, criteria diagnostically, and course biologically. Am J Dermatopathol. 2003;25(3):223–38.
14. Lange JR, Palis BE, Chang DC, Soong SJ, Balch CM. Melanoma in children and teenagers: an analysis of patients from the National Cancer Data Base. J Clin Oncol. 2007;25(11):1363–8.
15. Spitz S. Melanomas of childhood. Am J Pathol. 1948;24(3):591–609.
16. Pedrosa AF, Lopes JM, Azevedo F, Mota A. Spitz/Reed nevi: a review of clinical-dermatoscopic and histological correlation. Dermatol Pract Concept. 2016;6(2):37–41.
17. Tlougan BE, Orlow SJ, Schaffer JV. Spitz nevi: beliefs, behaviors, and experiences of pediatric dermatologists. JAMA Dermatol. 2013;149(3):283–91.
18. Requena C, Requena L, Kutzner H, Sánchez YE. Spitz nevus: a clinicopathological study of 349 cases. Am J Dermatopathol. 2009;31(2):107–16.
19. Weedon D, Little JH. Spindle and epithelioid cell nevi in children and adults. A review of 211 cases of the spitz nevus. Cancer. 1977;40(1):217–25.
20. Luo S, Sepehr A, Tsao H. Spitz nevi and other Spitzoid lesions: part I. Background and diagnoses. J Am Acad Dermatol. 2011;65(6):1073–84.
21. Luo S, Sepehr A, Tsao H. Spitz nevi and other Spitzoid lesions: part II. Natural history and management. J Am Acad Dermatol. 2011;65(6):1087–92.
22. Vollmer RT. Patient age in Spitz Nevus and malignant melanoma: implication of Bayes rule for differential diagnosis. Am J Clin Pathol. 2004;121(6):872–7.
23. Barnhill RL. The Spitzoid lesion: rethinking Spitz tumors, atypical variants, 'Spitzoid melanoma' and risk assessment. Mod Pathol. 2006;19:21–33.
24. Gelbard SN, Tripp JM, Marghoob AA, Kopf AW, Koenig KL, Kim JY, et al. Management of Spitz nevi: a survey of dermatologists in the United States. J Am Acad Dermatol. 2002;47(2):224–30.
25. Casso EM, Grin-Jorgensen CM, Grant-Kels JM. Spitz nevi. J Am Acad Dermatol. 1992;27(6):901–13.
26. Nino M, Brunetti B, Delfino S, Brunetti B, Panariello L, Russo D. Spitz Nevus: follow-up study of 8 cases of childhood starburst type and proposal for management. Dermatology. 2008;218(1):48–51.
27. Brunetti B, Nino M, Sammarco E, Scalvenzi M. Spitz naevus: a proposal for management. J Eur Acad Dermatol Venereol. 2005;19(3):391–3.
28. Hawryluk EB, Liang MG. Pediatric melanoma, moles, and sun safety. Pediatr Clin N Am. 2014;61(2):279–91.
29. Ludgate MW, Fullen DR, Lee J, Lowe L, Bradford C, Geiger J, et al. The atypical Spitz tumor of uncertain biologic potential. Cancer. 2009;115(3):631–41.
30. Vourch-Jourdain M, Martin L, Barbarot S. Large congenital melanocytic nevi: therapeutic management and melanoma risk: a systematic review. J Am Acad Dermatol. 2013;68(3):493–8.
31. Moscarella E, Piccolo V, Argenziano G, Lallas A, Longo C, Castagnetti F, et al. Problematic lesions in children. Dermatol Clin. 2013;31(4):535–47.

32. Krengel S, Hauschild A, Schäfer T. Melanoma risk in congenital melanocytic naevi: a systematic review. Br J Dermatol. 2006;155(1):1–8.
33. Slutsky JB, Barr JM, Femia AN, Marghoob AA. Large congenital melanocytic nevi: associated risks and management considerations. Semin Cutan Med Surg. 2010;29(2):79–84.
34. Marghoob AA, Schoenbach SP, Kopf AW, Orlow SJ, Nossa R, Bart RS. Large congenital melanocytic nevi and the risk for the development of malignant melanoma: a prospective study. Arch Dermatol. 1996;132(2):170–5.
35. Psaty EL, Scope A, Halpern AC, Marghoob AA. Defining the patient at high risk for melanoma. Int J Dermatol. 2010;49(4):362–76.
36. Berg P, Wennberg AM, Tuominen R, Sander B, Rozell BL, Platz A, et al. Germline CDKN2A mutations are rare in child and adolescent cutaneous melanoma. Melanoma Res. 2004;14(4):251.
37. Rigel DS. Epidemiology of melanoma. Semin Cutan Med Surg. 2010;29(4):204–9.
38. Boniol M, Autier P, Boyle P, Gandini S. Cutaneous melanoma attributable to sunbed use: systematic review and meta-analysis. BMJ. 2012;345:e4757.
39. Han D, Zager JS, Han G, Marzban SS, Puleo CA, Sarnaik AA, et al. The unique clinical characteristics of melanoma diagnosed in children. Ann Surg Oncol. 2012;19(12):3888–95.
40. Paradela S, Fonseca E, Pita-Fernández S, Kantrow SM, Diwan AH, Herzog C, et al. Prognostic factors for melanoma in children and adolescents: a clinicopathologic, single-center study of 137 patients. Cancer. 2010;116(18):4334–44.
41. Bartenstein DW, Kelleher CM, Friedmann AM, Duncan LM, Tsao H, Sober AJ, et al. Contrasting features of childhood and adolescent melanomas. Pediatr Dermatol. 2018;35(3):354–60.
42. Livestro DP, Kaine EM, Michaelson JS, Mihm MC, Haluska FG, Muzikansky A, et al. Melanoma in the young: differences and similarities with adult melanoma. Cancer. 2007;110(3):614–24.
43. Saenz NC, Saenz-Badillos J, Busam K, LaQuaglia MP, Corbally M, Brady MS. Childhood melanoma survival. Cancer. 1999;85(3):750–4.
44. Daryanani D, Plukker JT, Nap RE, Kuiper H, Hoekstra HJ. Adolescent melanoma: risk factors and long term survival. Eur J Surg Oncol J Eur Soc Surg Oncol Br Assoc Surg Oncol. 2006;32(2):218–23.
45. Leman JA, Evans A, Mooi W, MacKie RM. Outcomes and pathological review of a cohort of children with melanoma. Br J Dermatol. 2005;152(6):1321–3.
46. Moscarella E, Zalaudek I, Cerroni L, Sperduti I, Catricalà C, Smolle J, et al. Excised melanocytic lesions in children and adolescents - a 10-year survey. Br J Dermatol. 2012;167(2):368–73.
47. Pampena R, Piccolo V, Muscianese M, Kyrgidis A, Lai M, Russo T, et al. Melanoma in children: a systematic review and individual patient meta-analysis. J Eur Acad Dermatol Venereol. 2023;37(9):1758–76.
48. Parsons BG, Hay JL, Aspinwall LG, Zaugg K, Zhu A, Mooney RH, et al. Understanding skin screening practices among children at elevated risk for melanoma to inform interventions for melanoma prevention and control. J Cancer Educ. 2020;35(3):509.
49. Berk DR, LaBuz E, Dadras SS, Johnson DL, Swetter SM. Melanoma and melanocytic tumors of uncertain malignant potential in children, adolescents and young adults—the Stanford experience 1995–2008. Pediatr Dermatol. 2010;27(3):244–54.
50. Sondak VK, Taylor JMG, Sabel MS, Wang Y, Lowe L, Grover AC, et al. Mitotic rate and younger age are predictors of sentinel lymph node positivity: lessons learned from the generation of a probabilistic model. Ann Surg Oncol. 2004;11(3):247–58.

Melanoma and Pregnancy

Introduction

Although melanoma is more common in older individuals, it is the most common among malignancies associated with pregnancies. Pregnancy-associated melanoma (PAM) is loosely defined as any melanoma diagnosis between the onset of pregnancy until 1–5 years postpartum [1, 2]. The impact of pregnancy on melanoma and that of melanoma on pregnancy has been an area of controversy since case reports suggesting a relationship from the 1950s [3]. This is thought to be due to the immunologic changes in pregnancy, and these changes are analogous to the processes that allow for tolerance of cancer cells. Regulatory T cells (Tregs) are essential in suppressing the immune system to allow the fetus to survive [4]. Furthermore, the maternal-fetal interface has a Th2 predominance, similar to the immunologic state in malignancy [5]. Despite these similarities, there is no compelling evidence to treat PAM differently from melanoma in a nonpregnant individual.

Melanoma During Pregnancy

A diagnosis of melanoma during pregnancy does not appear to be associated with a poorer prognosis than in nonpregnant controls. A retrospective cohort study using data from the Swedish National and Regional Registries compared 185 women with PAM to 5348 women of similar age and found no statistically significant difference in overall survival (log-rank χ^2 1[r] = 0.84, P − 0.361) [6]. A multivariate cox analysis in the same study also found that pregnancy status at time of melanoma diagnosis was not related to survival (hazard ratio 1.08 for death in pregnant group, 95% CI: 0.60–1.93) [6]. A large population-based cohort study from the Swedish Cancer and Multi-Generation Register found that among 6857 women with cutaneous melanoma, 1019 of whom were classified as having PAM, cause-specific mortality was not statistically significant (hazard ratio 1.09, 95% CI: 0.83–1.42) [7]. Similarly, a large population-based study in California of pregnant women with melanoma

© The Author(s), under exclusive license to Springer Nature Switzerland AG 2024
S. Ortiz-Urda et al., *Melanoma*, https://doi.org/10.1007/978-3-031-59128-0_9

found no evidence of a more advanced stage, thicker tumors, increased metastases to lymph nodes, or worsened survival [8].

However, one cancer registry study in Norway found that the diagnosis of melanoma during pregnancy was associated with a slightly increased cause-specific death (HR 1.52, 95% CI: 1.01–2.31, $p = 0.047$) [9]. Therefore, it is unclear whether there is an impact of pregnancy on risk of mortality from melanoma.

Treatment for Patients with Advanced PAM

Multidisciplinary counseling is necessary to manage safety for both the mother and fetus. Wide local excision can be carried out in all trimesters under local anesthesia, with sentinel lymph node biopsy under general anesthesia performed in the postpartum period [10].

Currently used anesthetic agents do not have teratogenic effects, but there may be increased risk to the mother with deep venous thromboses, hypotension secondary to compression of the IVC from the gravid uterus, and risk of aspiration from decreased lower esophageal sphincter tone [11].

Given the immunosuppressive changes in pregnancy to support immune tolerance of the developing fetus, one may expect that immune checkpoint inhibitor therapy may increase the risk of compromising the fetus. Animal studies have shown that anti-PD-1 or anti-PD-L1 therapy increases the risk of spontaneous abortions [12, 13]. The FDA categorizes anti-PD-1 agents as pregnancy category D, whereas ipilimumab is pregnancy category C (possibly from a less clear role of CTLA-4 in fetal immune tolerance) [14]. One case report of nivolumab use for 14 months until the patient was found to be 7 weeks pregnant prompted discontinuation of nivolumab and led to an uneventful pregnancy for the mother, but the fetus did suffer from intrauterine growth restriction and congenital hypothyroidism before reaching appropriate weight and milestones [15]. Another case report describes an 18-week pregnant patient with metastatic melanoma who tolerated two cycles of nivolumab and ipilimumab, but the treatment did not slow tumor progression [16].

Because the MAPK pathway is crucial for the developing fetus, the use of BRAF/MEK inhibitors in pregnant patients with melanoma requires thorough discussion and consideration. Among BRAF inhibitors, there is evidence from animal studies that dabrafenib is teratogenic, but vemurafenib does not cross the placenta [17]. In one case study, a 37-year-old woman with BRAF-mutant melanoma during the second trimester of pregnancy started vemurafenib but died 2.5 months later, while the fetus was delivered prematurely because of growth restriction [18]. Another case report describes a 36-year-old woman who developed widespread metastases during her 7th week of a twin pregnancy prompting vemurafenib treatment but after 1 month was complicated by toxic epidermal necrolysis with over 70% body surface area involvement [19]. The evidence of systemic therapy in pregnancy remains sparse and effects are not well understood.

Melanoma During the Postpartum Period

Similar to the pregnant state, the cohort study based on the Swedish Cancer and Multi-Generation register found no evidence of worse prognosis of melanoma diagnosed in the postpartum period [7]. However, one English cancer registry that examined the relationship between gestation and childbirth with cancer found an increased rate of mortality in the first year postpartum but not in the second through fifth years postpartum [20]. One population-based study found that the observed rates of cancer were lower than expected during pregnancy and rebounded after delivery [21]. This observation may be due to a rebound effect whereby the melanoma diagnosis is delayed [21].

Melanoma Diagnosed Prior to Pregnancy

One meta-analysis of five studies found no significant effect of a subsequent pregnancy on melanoma mortality [22]. However, it is recommended to consider delaying pregnancy by 2–3 years in patients with poor prognostic factors because most cancer recurrences occur during this time and pregnancy may increase the risks of systemic therapy. The overall risk of metastatic disease involving the fetus is low unless there is widely metastatic disease [3].

Influence of Hormones on Melanoma

One meta-analysis of 3796 cases of melanoma in women with previous oral contraceptive pills (OCP) use and 9442 controls with no history of OCP use demonstrated no increased risk of melanoma (pooled OR 0.95, 95% CI: 0.87–1.04) [23]. A review of the relationship between OCP use and the development of skin cancer found no significantly increased risk [24]. A prospective cohort study of French women found a nonsignificant positive association between OCP use and melanoma risk, but that OCP use was also positively associated with other known risk factors such as history of suntan bed use and sunburns [25]. Hormone replacement therapy appears to be like OCPs in melanoma risk. One review of 12 studies found that ten demonstrated no association between hormone replacement therapy and melanoma risk [26].

References

1. Holtan SG, Creedon DJ, Haluska P, Markovic SN. Cancer and pregnancy: parallels in growth, invasion, and immune modulation and implications for cancer therapeutic agents. Mayo Clin Proc. 2009;84(11):985–1000.
2. Todd SP, Driscoll MS. Prognosis for women diagnosed with melanoma during, before, or after pregnancy: weighing the evidence. Int J Womens Dermatol. 2017;3(1):26–9.

3. Driscoll MS, Grant-Kels JM. Hormones, nevi, and melanoma: an approach to the patient. J Am Acad Dermatol. 2007;57(6):919–31; quiz 932–6.
4. Leber A, Teles A, Zenclussen AC. Regulatory T cells and their role in pregnancy. Am J Reprod Immunol. 2010;63(6):445–59.
5. Nevala WK, Vachon CM, Leontovich AA, Scott CG, Thompson MA, Markovic SN, et al. Evidence of systemic Th2-driven chronic inflammation in patients with metastatic melanoma. Clin Cancer Res. 2009;15(6):1931–9.
6. Lens MB, Rosdahl I, Ahlbom A, Farahmand BY, Synnerstad I, Boeryd B, et al. Effect of pregnancy on survival in women with cutaneous malignant melanoma. J Clin Oncol. 2004;22(21):4369–75.
7. Johansson ALV, Andersson TML, Plym A, Ullenhag GJ, Møller H, Lambe M. Mortality in women with pregnancy-associated malignant melanoma. J Am Acad Dermatol. 2014;71(6):1093–101.
8. O'Meara AT, Cress R, Xing G, Danielsen B, Smith LH. Malignant melanoma in pregnancy. A population-based evaluation. Cancer. 2005;103(6):1217–26.
9. Stensheim H, Møller B, van Dijk T, Fosså SD. Cause-specific survival for women diagnosed with cancer during pregnancy or lactation: a registry-based cohort study. J Clin Oncol. 2009;27(1):45–51.
10. Broer N, Buonocore S, Goldberg C, Truini C, Faries MB, Narayan D, et al. A proposal for the timing of management of patients with melanoma presenting during pregnancy. J Surg Oncol. 2012;106(1):36–40.
11. Cheek TG, Baird E. Anesthesia for nonobstetric surgery: maternal and fetal considerations. Clin Obstet Gynecol. 2009;52(4):535–45.
12. D'Addio F, Riella LV, Mfarrej BG, Chabtini L, Adams LT, Yeung M, et al. The link between the PDL1 costimulatory pathway and Th17 in fetomaternal tolerance. J Immunol. 2011;187(9):4530–41.
13. Poulet FM, Wolf JJ, Herzyk DJ, DeGeorge JJ. An evaluation of the impact of PD-1 pathway blockade on reproductive safety of therapeutic PD-1 inhibitors. Birth Defects Res B Dev Reprod Toxicol. 2016;107(2):108–19.
14. Johnson DB, Sullivan RJ, Menzies AM. Immune checkpoint inhibitors in challenging populations. Cancer. 2017;123(11):1904–11.
15. Xu W, Moor RJ, Walpole ET, Atkinson VG. Pregnancy with successful foetal and maternal outcome in a melanoma patient treated with nivolumab in the first trimester: case report and review of the literature. Melanoma Res. 2019;29(3):333–7.
16. Menzer C, Beedgen B, Rom J, Duffert CM, Volckmar AL, Sedlaczek O, et al. Immunotherapy with ipilimumab plus nivolumab in a stage IV melanoma patient during pregnancy. Eur J Cancer. 1990;2018(104):239–42.
17. Grunewald S, Jank A. New systemic agents in dermatology with respect to fertility, pregnancy, and lactation. J Dtsch Dermatol Ges J Ger Soc Dermatol. 2015;13(4):277–89. quiz 290
18. Maleka A, Enblad G, Sjörs G, Lindqvist A, Ullenhag GJ. Treatment of metastatic malignant melanoma with vemurafenib during pregnancy. J Clin Oncol. 2013;31(11):192–3.
19. de Haan J, van Thienen JV, Casaer M, Hannivoort RA, Van Calsteren K, van Tuyl M, et al. Severe adverse reaction to vemurafenib in a pregnant woman with metastatic melanoma. Case Rep Oncol. 2018;11(1):119–24.
20. Møller H, Purushotham A, Linklater KM, Garmo H, Holmberg L, Lambe M, et al. Recent childbirth is an adverse prognostic factor in breast cancer and melanoma, but not in Hodgkin lymphoma. Eur J Cancer. 2013;49(17):3686–93.
21. Andersson TML, Johansson ALV, Fredriksson I, Lambe M. Cancer during pregnancy and the postpartum period: a population-based study. Cancer. 2015;121(12):2072–7.
22. Byrom L, Olsen CM, Knight L, Khosrotehrani K, Green AC. Does pregnancy after a diagnosis of melanoma affect prognosis? Systematic review and meta-analysis. Dermatologic Surg. 2015;41(8):875–82.
23. Gefeller O, Hassan K, Wille L. Cutaneous malignant melanoma in women and the role of oral contraceptives. Br J Dermatol. 1998;138(1):122–4.

24. Leslie KK, Espey E. Oral contraceptives and skin cancer: is there a link? Am J Clin Dermatol. 2005;6(6):349–55.
25. Cervenka I, Mahamat-Saleh Y, Savoye I, Dartois L, Boutron-Ruault MC, Fournier A, et al. Oral contraceptive use and cutaneous melanoma risk: a French prospective cohort study. Int J Cancer. 2018;143(10):2390–9.
26. Gupta A, Driscoll MS. Do hormones influence melanoma? Facts and controversies. Clin Dermatol. 2010;28(3):287–92.

Mucosal Melanoma 10

Although melanocytes are well known for its role in producing melanin to protect our skin from damage caused by UV radiation, melanocytes may have other important roles. In mucosal tissues, where UV radiation is less likely, melanocytes are thought to be involved in immunity. Mucosal melanocytes supply melanin to these important immunologic areas for antimicrobial defense [1]. Since mucosal melanocytes are not typically exposed to UV radiation, the pathogenesis to melanoma is unknown. No clear risk factors have been identified, but there is an increased risk of developing vulvovaginal and anorectal mucosal melanoma in those with a family history of cutaneous melanoma [2]. Studies have not shown any association of human papilloma viruses, human herpes viruses, and polyomavirus with mucosal melanoma pathogenesis [3–5].

Mucosal melanomas represent only about 1.4% of all melanomas [6]. Unlike cutaneous melanomas that have seen increasing incidence over recent years, the incidence of mucosal melanomas has been stable [3]. Mucosal melanomas are more common in Caucasians than in other racial groups [7]. However, because cutaneous melanomas are much rarer in non-Caucasians, mucosal melanomas represent a larger proportion of all melanomas in non-Caucasians [7]. The age of diagnosis for mucosal melanoma (median age 70) is greater than for cutaneous melanomas (median age 55) [8].

While mucosal melanoma can arise in any mucosal epithelium, the majority are head and neck (31–55% of cases), vulvovaginal (18–40% of cases), and anorectal (17–24% of cases) [6, 8]. Sometimes, mucosal melanomas are divided by region: an upper region consisting of the oral cavity, nasal cavity, and upper GI tract and a lower region consisting of the lower GI tract, anorectum, and genitalia. There is a female predominance of mucosal melanomas in the United States (2.8 cases per million per year) compared to males (1.5 per million per year) due to substantially higher rates of genital tract melanomas in females [6].

Mucosal melanomas are often diagnosed at later stages because they are often concealed. Diagnosis is also complicated by the observation that an amelanotic appearance is common among mucosal lesions. Locoregional nodal metastasis at diagnosis is common, with 21% of head and neck, 23% of vulvovaginal, and 61% of anorectal mucosal melanomas presenting with involved lymph nodes [9]. Patients diagnosed with metastatic mucosal melanoma have lower median survival (9.1 months from time of metastasis) than patients diagnosed with metastatic melanoma of other subtypes of the same stage (13.4 months for uveal melanoma and 11.7 months for cutaneous melanoma) [10]. Considering all stages of mucosal melanoma, the 5-year survival is 16–27%, compared to about 80% for cutaneous melanoma [11].

Head and Neck

The head and neck region is the most common site for mucosal melanoma in men and second most common site in women [12]. The overall survival rates for head and neck mucosal melanomas are 43% at 2 years and 18% at 5 years [13]. Fifty-six percent of head and neck mucosal melanomas are sinonasal in location, whereas 41% were in the oral cavity [14]. In a study of 328 cases of mucosal melanoma in the sinonasal tract, 81% occurred in the nasal cavity, of which the most common sites are the septum and lateral wall [15]. Nasal cavity melanomas have a better prognosis (5-year survival 31%) than melanoma arising in the sinuses (5-year survival 0%) [16]. Common presenting symptoms for sinonasal tract mucosal melanomas were epistaxis (45%), mass lesion (37%), and/or nasal obstruction (30%) [16].

Oral and oropharyngeal primary mucosal melanoma tumors more frequently present with regional metastases (44%) than primary tumors of the sinonasal tract (11%) [13]. Oral mucosal melanomas arise most commonly at the hard palate and maxillary gingiva [17]. The 5-year survival for oral melanoma is roughly 15% [17]. These tumors are usually asymptomatic, but later, symptoms can include ulceration, bleeding, pain, and loose teeth [17]. Differential diagnoses of oral melanoma include melanosis, oral nevi, melanotic macule, smoking-associated melanosis, post-inflammatory pigmentation medication-related pigmentation, melanoacanthoma, amalgam tattoo, and Kaposi's sarcoma [17, 18].

Genitourinary

The incidence of genitourinary melanomas is much greater in women than in men (1.74 cases per million person-years vs. 0.17 cases per million person-years, respectively) [19]. In women, 77% of mucosal melanoma arise in the vulva, 5–20% in the vagina, and few arise elsewhere, primarily at the cervix [20]. Vulvovaginal melanoma has a 5-year overall survival rate of 36%, with better survival for vulvar melanoma than for vaginal melanoma (53% vs. 15%, respectively) [19]. The most common sites are the clitoral area (30.8%) and labia majora (27.3%), followed by the labia minora (19.2%) and periurethral area (11.3%), and the vaginal introitus (4.0%) is least common [21]. Presenting symptoms include vaginal bleeding (80%), discharge (25%), palpable mass (15%), and pain (10%) [22].

Anorectal

The vast majority of anorectal melanomas (96%) are within 6 cm from the anal rim, since melanocytes are found mostly in the anal squamous zone, sporadically in the anal transition zone, and not in the colorectal zone [23, 24]. The average age of diagnosis is 71 years, and the incidence of anorectal melanoma may be increasing similarly to cutaneous melanoma [25]. The most common presentations are rectal bleeding, anorectal pain, changes in bowel habits, and sensation of mass [26]. Nearly two thirds of anorectal melanomas are misdiagnosed, most often as hemorrhoids, adenocarcinoma, polyps, and rectal cancer [23]. Patients with anorectal melanoma misdiagnosed as hemorrhoids have particularly poor prognosis with a 1-year survival of 29% [23].

Molecular Biology of Mucosal Melanoma

While cutaneous melanoma may have among the highest rates of single nucleotide variants of any cancer, mucosal melanomas have on average tenfold fewer single nucleotide variants and are not characterized by UV mutational signatures [27]. However, mucosal melanomas have a much higher rate of copy number and structural variants compared to cutaneous melanoma (average of 361 per tumor vs. 97 per tumor, respectively) [27].

In contrast to cutaneous melanomas, of which the majority have activating mutations in BRAF or NRAS, only about 5% of mucosal melanomas have BRAF-activating mutations and about 14% have NRAS-activating mutations [28–30]. Some subtypes may have a higher proportion of NRAS mutations, such as vaginal melanomas that have a 43% NRAS mutation rate, and this is associated with a worse overall survival among vaginal melanomas [31]. Amplifications and activating mutations in KIT are observed at higher rates of 14–39% in mucosal melanomas [29].

Neurofibromin 1 functions as a tumor suppressor by acting as a negative regulator of Ras. A meta-analysis of mutations in mucosal melanoma found that NF1 is mutated at a rate of 14%, which is similar to the rate in cutaneous melanoma from the TCGA cohort [30]. SPRED1 (sprout-related EVH1 domain containing protein 1) recruits NF1 to the plasma membrane to convert active Ras-GTP to the inactive Ras-GDP. Therefore, SPRED1 also functions as a tumor suppressor and is diminished in some mucosal melanoma either by deep deletion or by a truncating mutation combined with loss of the wild-type SPRED1 allele [30]. Both NF1 and SPRED1 may be involved in tumor progression in mucosal melanoma and future studies may demonstrate how it can affect prognosis and treatment.

SF3B1 is the most frequently mutated spliceosome gene in cancers and mutations in this protein lead to dysregulated RNA processing and subsequent tumorigenesis [32]. Mutations of SF3B1 in mucosal melanoma are almost exclusively at the R625 residue, whereas in other cancers, such as hematologic malignancies and breast cancer, mutations are more common at the K666 and K700 residues [30].

Mucosal melanomas with SF3B1 mutations were found to be associated with shorter overall survival (34.9 months vs. 79.9 months in wild-type) and progression-free survival (16.9 months vs. 35.7 months in wild-type) [33].

In a whole-genome sequencing study in a cohort of oral mucosal melanomas, authors found that structural variants such as a translocation between chromosome 5 and chromosome 12 had significantly worse median overall survival (9.0 vs. 28.0 months without the translocation) [34]. These authors also found amplifications in KIT, CDK4, TERT, NOTCH2, and CCND1, along with losses in CDKN2A/B and TP53 in oral mucosal melanomas [34]. Future studies may suggest assessing mucosal melanomas for structural variants to better estimate prognosis.

Management of Primary Disease

Complete surgical resection offers the greatest likelihood of disease cure, but wide negative margins are often difficult to achieve because of the lentiginous growth pattern, multifocal nature, and anatomical constraints [9]. Although surgery remains a mainstay in treatment, 50–90% of patients exhibit local recurrence [9]. Extensive surgery to achieve negative margins needs to be weighed with the operative morbidity and risk of recurrence [35]. Radiotherapy may be used as definitive treatment of unresectable, locally advanced mucosal melanoma, leading complete or partial responses in 29% and 58% of patients, respectively [36].

Adjuvant Therapy

Adjuvant radiation therapy after wide local excision can improve local control. For anorectal melanoma, 25–36 grays in 5–6 fractions delivered to extended fields and draining lymphatics following sphincter-sparing excision resulted in local control in 74–82% of cases [37]. However, there remained high rates of metastasis, leading to a 5-year overall survival rate of 30% [37]. Patients who received extended-field radiotherapy had higher rates of lymphedema without benefit in local control, lymph node control, or overall survival compared to patients who received limited-field radiotherapy [37].

Having once been standard of care, traditional chemotherapy is now much less used. One study showed that a group treated with chemotherapy of temozolomide plus cisplatin had 20.8 months of survival, which was significantly greater than 9.4 months for the interferon-treated group and 5.4 months for the observation groups [38]. Other studies have shown some efficacy of chemotherapy in mucosal melanoma and increased overall survival with adjuvant chemotherapy [39–42]. However, promising results of systemic targeted therapy or immune checkpoint inhibitors suggest that they may be effectively used in the adjuvant setting [43, 44].

Systemic Therapy

Advances in immunotherapy and the identification of genetic alterations in mucosal melanoma have yielded promising therapeutics. The finding of activating mutations and amplifications in KIT in some mucosal melanomas have led to trials of KIT inhibitors: imatinib, nilotinib, sorafenib, dasatinib, and sunitinib [45–49]. In a study to identify which KIT mutation types are most susceptible to KIT-targeted therapy in 25 KIT mutant mucosal melanoma patients, all 6 of 6 patients who had a partial, durable, or complete response had tumors with a L576P or K642E mutation [45]. This suggests that specific mutations confer greater oncogenic driver capacity and may be an indicator of sensitivity to KIT inhibitors [45]. A clinical trial demonstrated that one cohort with KIT mutant mucosal melanomas that were refractory to previous imatinib treatment and subsequently received nilotinib treatment led to 3 out of 11 patients achieving disease control at 4 months [46]. Two patients with either a L576P or K642E KIT mutation achieved durable partial responses to nilotinib, demonstrating that nilotinib can have clinical effect in overcoming resistance to imatinib [46].

Immune checkpoint blockade with anti-CTLA-4 or anti-PD-1/PD-L1 agents has drastically changed the treatability of cutaneous melanoma, and mucosal melanomas also seem to respond albeit at lower rates. One study of 71 patients with metastatic mucosal melanoma treated with ipilimumab in Italy reported a response rate of 12%, median progression-free survival of 4.3 months, and median overall survival of 6.4 months [50]. Anti-PD-1 treatment may yield an increased overall response rate (35%) and progression-free survival (5 months) [51, 52]. A retrospective multicenter study evaluating the efficacy of anti-PD-1 agents in 35 patients with mucosal melanoma showed partial responses in 8 (23%), stable disease in 7 (20%), and no patients with complete responses [53]. The median progression-free survival was 3.9 months and median overall survival was 12.4 months [53].

A pooled analysis of phase III clinical trials comparing immunotherapy responses found that the combination of anti-PD-1 and anti-CTLA-4 yielded a greater objective response rate of 37.1%, compared to 23.3% for anti-PD-1 monotherapy and 8.3% for anti-CTLA-4 monotherapy in mucosal melanoma [54]. Some studies are also evaluating the combination of radiotherapy and immune checkpoint inhibitors or of chemotherapy with immune checkpoint inhibitors [55–57].

The guidelines from ASCO for systemic treatment of mucosal melanoma state that without additional data, patients with unresectable or metastatic mucosal melanoma may be offered treatment options like unresectable or metastatic cutaneous melanoma [58]. Therefore, patients may be offered first-line treatment with anti-PD-1 monotherapy or combination with ipilimumab, and if their melanoma carries a BRAF V600 mutation, they may be treated with BRAF/MEK combination inhibitor therapy [58].

References

1. Mackintosh JA. The antimicrobial properties of melanocytes, melanosomes and melanin and the evolution of black skin. J Theor Biol. 2001;211(2):101–13.
2. Cazenave H, Maubec E, Mohamdi H, Grange F, Bressac-de Paillerets B, Demenais F, et al. Genital and anorectal mucosal melanoma is associated with cutaneous melanoma in patients and in families. Br J Dermatol. 2013;169(3):594–9.
3. Dahlgren L, Schedvins K, Kanter-Lewensohn L, Dalianis T, Ragnarsson-Olding BK. Human papilloma virus (HPV) is rarely detected in malignant melanomas of sun sheltered mucosal membranes. Acta Oncol. 2005;44(7):694–9.
4. Lundberg R, Brytting M, Dahlgren L, Kanter-Lewensohn L, Schloss L, Dalianis T, et al. Human herpes virus DNA is rarely detected in non-UV light-associated primary malignant melanomas of mucous membranes. Anticancer Res. 2006;26(5B):3627–31.
5. Giraud G, Ramqvist T, Ragnarsson-Olding B, Dalianis T. DNA from BK Virus and JC virus and from KI, WU, and MC polyomaviruses as well as from simian virus 40 is not detected in non-UV-light-associated primary malignant melanomas of mucous membranes. J Clin Microbiol. 2008;46(11):3595–8.
6. McLaughlin CC, Wu X-C, Jemal A, Martin HJ, Roche LM, Chen VW. Incidence of noncutaneous melanomas in the US. Cancer. 2005;103(5):1000–7.
7. Mihajlovic M, Vlajkovic S, Jovanovic P, Stefanovic V. Primary mucosal melanomas: a comprehensive review. Int J Clin Exp Pathol. 2012;5(8):739–53.
8. Chang AE, Karnell LH, Menck HR. The National Cancer Data Base report on cutaneous and noncutaneous melanoma: a summary of 84,836 cases from the past decade. The American College of Surgeons Commission on Cancer and the American Cancer Society. Cancer. 1998;83(8):1664–78.
9. Carvajal RD, Spencer SA, Lydiatt W. Mucosal melanoma: a clinically and biologically unique disease entity. J Natl Compr Cancer Netw. 2012;10(3):345–56.
10. Postow MA, Kuk D, Bogatch K, Carvajal RD. Assessment of overall survival from time of metastasis in mucosal, uveal, and cutaneous melanoma. J Clin Oncol. 2014;32(15):9074–4.
11. Lian B, Cui CL, Zhou L, Song X, Zhang XS, Wu D, et al. The natural history and patterns of metastases from mucosal melanoma: an analysis of 706 prospectively-followed patients. Ann Oncol. 2017;28(4):868–73.
12. Lerner BA, Stewart LA, Horowitz DP, Carvajal RD. Mucosal melanoma: new insights and therapeutic options for a unique and aggressive disease. Oncologia. 2017;31(11):23–32.
13. Plavc G, But-Hadžić J, Aničin A, Lanišnik B, Didanović V, Strojan P. Mucosal melanoma of the head and neck: a population-based study from Slovenia, 1985-2013. Radiat Oncol. 2016;11(1):137.
14. Patel SG, Prasad ML, Escrig M, Singh B, Shaha AR, Kraus DH, et al. Primary mucosal malignant melanoma of the head and neck. Head Neck. 2002;24(3):247–57.
15. Manolidis S, Donald PJ. Malignant mucosal melanoma of the head and neck. Cancer. 1997;80(8):1373–86.
16. Thompson LDR, Wieneke JA, Miettinen M. Sinonasal tract and nasopharyngeal melanomas: a clinicopathologic study of 115 cases with a proposed staging system. Am J Surg Pathol. 2003;27(5):594–611.
17. Hicks MJ, Flaitz CM. Oral mucosal melanoma: epidemiology and pathobiology. Oral Oncol. 2000;36(2):152–69.
18. Patrick RJ, Fenske NA, Messina JL. Primary mucosal melanoma. J Am Acad Dermatol. 2007;56(5):828–34.
19. Vyas R, Thompson CL, Zargar H, Selph J, Gerstenblith MR. Epidemiology of genitourinary melanoma in the United States: 1992 through 2012. J Am Acad Dermatol. 2016;75(1):144–50.
20. Weinstock MA. Malignant melanoma of the vulva and vagina in the United States: patterns of incidence and population-based estimates of survival. Am J Obstet Gynecol. 1994;171(5):1225–30.

21. Ragnarsson-Olding BK, Nilsson BR, Kanter-Lewensohn LR, Lagerlöf B, Ringborg UK. Malignant melanoma of the vulva in a nationwide, 25-year study of 219 Swedish females. Cancer. 1999;86(7):1285–93.
22. Terzakis E, Androutsopoulos G, Adonakis G, Zygouris D, Grigoriadis C, Decavalas G. Vaginal primary malignant melanoma: report of four cases and review of the literature. Eur J Gynaecol Oncol. 2011;32(1):122–4.
23. Zhang S, Gao F, Wan D. Effect of misdiagnosis on the prognosis of anorectal malignant melanoma. J Cancer Res Clin Oncol. 2010;136(9):1401–5.
24. Clemmensen OJ, Fenger C. Melanocytes in the anal canal epithelium. Histopathology. 1991;18(3):237–41.
25. Coté TR, Sobin LH. Primary melanomas of the esophagus and anorectum: epidemiologic comparison with melanoma of the skin. Melanoma Res. 2009;19(1):58–60.
26. Chute DJ, Cousar JB, Mills SE. Anorectal malignant melanoma: morphologic and immunohistochemical features. Am J Clin Pathol. 2006;126(1):93–100.
27. Furney SJ, Turajlic S, Stamp G, Nohadani M, Carlisle A, Thomas JM, et al. Genome sequencing of mucosal melanomas reveals that they are driven by distinct mechanisms from cutaneous melanoma. J Pathol. 2013;230(3):261–9.
28. Curtin JA, Fridlyand J, Kageshita T, Patel HN, Busam KJ, Kutzner H, et al. Distinct sets of genetic alterations in melanoma. N Engl J Med. 2005;353(20):2135–47.
29. Curtin JA, Busam K, Pinkel D, Bastian BC. Somatic activation of KIT in distinct subtypes of melanoma. J Clin Oncol. 2006;24(26):4340–6.
30. Nassar KW, Tan AC. The mutational landscape of mucosal melanoma. Semin Cancer Biol. 2020;61:139–48.
31. Omholt K, Grafström E, Kanter-Lewensohn L, Hansson J, Ragnarsson-Olding BK. KIT pathway alterations in mucosal melanomas of the vulva and other sites. Clin Cancer Res. 2011;17(12):3933–42.
32. Darman RB, Seiler M, Agrawal AA, Lim KH, Peng S, Aird D, et al. Cancer-associated SF3B1 hotspot mutations induce cryptic 3′ splice site selection through use of a different branch point. Cell Rep. 2015;13(5):1033–45.
33. Quek C, Rawson RV, Ferguson PM, Shang P, Silva I, Saw RPM, et al. Recurrent hotspot SF3B1 mutations at codon 625 in vulvovaginal mucosal melanoma identified in a study of 27 Australian mucosal melanomas. Oncotarget. 2019;10(9):930–41.
34. Zhou R, Shi C, Tao W, Li J, Wu J, Han Y, et al. Analysis of mucosal melanoma whole-genome landscapes reveals clinically relevant genomic aberrations. Clin Cancer Res. 2019;25(12):3548–60.
35. Tyrrell H, Payne M. Combatting mucosal melanoma: recent advances and future perspectives. Melanoma Manage. 2018;5(3):MMT11.
36. Wada H, Nemoto K, Ogawa Y, Hareyama M, Yoshida H, Takamura A, et al. A multi-institutional retrospective analysis of external radiotherapy for mucosal melanoma of the head and neck in Northern Japan. Int J Radiat Oncol. 2004;59(2):495–500.
37. Kelly P, Zagars GK, Cormier JN, Ross MI, Guadagnolo BA. Sphincter-sparing local excision and hypofractionated radiation therapy for anorectal melanoma. Cancer. 2011;117(20):4747–55.
38. Lian B, Si L, Cui C, Chi Z, Sheng X, Mao L, et al. Phase II randomized trial comparing high dose IFN-α2b with temozolomide plus cisplatin as systemic adjuvant therapy for resected mucosal melanoma. Clin Cancer Res. 2013;19(16):4488–98.
39. Bartell HL, Bedikian AY, Papadopoulos NE, Dett TK, Ballo MT, Myers JN, et al. Biochemotherapy in patients with advanced head and neck mucosal melanoma. Head Neck. 2008;30(12):1592–8.
40. Harting MS, Kim KB. Biochemotherapy in patients with advanced vulvovaginal mucosal melanoma. Melanoma Res. 2004;14(6):517–20.
41. Kim KB, Sanguino AM, Hodges C, Papadopoulos NE, Eton O, Camacho LH, et al. Biochemotherapy in patients with metastatic anorectal mucosal melanoma. Cancer. 2004;100(7):1478–83.

42. Lai Y, Meng X, Liu Q, Lu H, Guo L, Wang S, et al. Impact of adjuvant therapy on survival for sinonasal mucosal melanoma. Acta Otolaryngol. 2020;140(1):79–84.
43. Petrella TM, Fletcher GG, Knight G, McWhirter E, Rajagopal S, Song X, et al. Systemic adjuvant therapy for adult patients at high risk for recurrent cutaneous or mucosal melanoma: an Ontario Health (Cancer Care Ontario) clinical practice guideline. Curr Oncol. 2020;27(1):43–52.
44. Baetz TD, Fletcher GG, Knight G, McWhirter E, Rajagopal S, Song X, et al. Systemic adjuvant therapy for adult patients at high risk for recurrent melanoma: a systematic review. Cancer Treat Rev. 2020;87:102032.
45. Carvajal RD, Antonescu CR, Wolchok JD, Chapman PB, Roman R-A, Teitcher J, et al. KIT as a therapeutic target in metastatic melanoma. JAMA. 2011;305(22):2327–34.
46. Carvajal RD, Lawrence DP, Weber JS, Gajewski TF, Gonzalez R, Lutzky J, et al. Phase II study of nilotinib in melanoma harboring KIT alterations following progression to prior KIT inhibition. Clin Cancer Res. 2015;21(10):2289–96.
47. Woodman SE, Trent JC, Stemke-Hale K, Lazar AJ, Pricl S, Pavan GM, et al. Activity of dasatinib against L576P KIT mutant melanoma: molecular, cellular, and clinical correlates. Mol Cancer Ther. 2009;8(8):2079–85.
48. Quintás-Cardama A, Lazar AJ, Woodman SE, Kim K, Ross M, Hwu P. Complete response of stage IV anal mucosal melanoma expressing KIT Val560Asp to the multikinase inhibitor sorafenib. Nat Clin Pract Oncol. 2008;5(12):737–40.
49. Minor DR, Kashani-Sabet M, Garrido M, O'Day SJ, Hamid O, Bastian BC. Sunitinib therapy for melanoma patients with KIT mutations. Clin Cancer Res. 2012;18(5):1457–63.
50. Del Vecchio M, Di Guardo L, Ascierto PA, Grimaldi AM, Sileni VC, Pigozzo J, et al. Efficacy and safety of ipilimumab 3 mg/kg in patients with pretreated, metastatic, mucosal melanoma. Eur J Cancer. 2014;50(1):121–7.
51. Moya-Plana A, Herrera Gómez RG, Rossoni C, Dercle L, Ammari S, Girault I, et al. Evaluation of the efficacy of immunotherapy for non-resectable mucosal melanoma. Cancer Immunol Immunother. 2019;68(7):1171–8.
52. Mignard C, Deschamps Huvier A, Gillibert A, Duval Modeste AB, Dutriaux C, Khammari A, et al. Efficacy of immunotherapy in patients with metastatic mucosal or uveal melanoma. J Oncol. 2018;2018:e1908065. Available from https://www.hindawi.com/journals/jo/2018/1908065/.
53. Shoushtari AN, Munhoz RR, Kuk D, Ott PA, Johnson DB, Tsai KK, et al. The efficacy of anti-PD-1 agents in acral and mucosal melanoma. Cancer. 2016;122(21):3354–62.
54. D'Angelo SP, Larkin J, Sosman JA, Lebbé C, Brady B, Neyns B, et al. Efficacy and safety of nivolumab alone or in combination with ipilimumab in patients with mucosal melanoma: a pooled analysis. J Clin Oncol. 2017;35(2):226–35.
55. Schiavone MB, Broach V, Shoushtari AN, Carvajal RD, Alektiar K, Kollmeier MA, et al. Combined immunotherapy and radiation for treatment of mucosal melanomas of the lower genital tract. Gynecol Oncol Rep. 2016;16:42–6.
56. Escorcia FE, Postow MA, Barker CA. Radiotherapy and immune checkpoint blockade for melanoma: a promising combinatorial strategy in need of further investigation. Cancer J Sudbury Mass. 2017;23(1):32–9.
57. Apetoh L, Ladoire S, Coukos G, Ghiringhelli F. Combining immunotherapy and anticancer agents: the right path to achieve cancer cure? Ann Oncol. 2015;26(9):1813–23.
58. Seth R, Messersmith H, Kaur V, Kirkwood JM, Kudchadkar R, McQuade JL, et al. Systemic therapy for melanoma: ASCO guideline. J Clin Oncol. 2020;38(33):3947–70.

Uveal Melanoma

11

Uveal melanoma (UM) affects uveal tissues of the eye—namely, the iris, ciliary body, and, most commonly, the choroid (90%) [1]. Its clinical and pathologic features are unique, including virtually exclusive metastasis to the liver in high-risk cases. Although it accounts for only about 5% of all melanomas, it is the most common primary intraocular malignancy in adults [2]. Risk factors for UM include light skin color, cutaneous freckles and nevi, red or blond hair, and light-colored irides [3–5]. Given these risk factors, the incidence rate is between 8 and 196 times greater in light-skinned non-Hispanic Caucasians than in individuals of African, Asian, or Hispanic descent [2, 6–9]. Unlike in cutaneous melanoma, rates of UM have not increased over the past several decades in response to increased UV light exposure [10]. The incidence of UM is slightly greater in males than in females [8, 11], but this difference may be due to a significantly increased rate in males 65 years old or older [9]. Peak incidence also occurs almost a decade earlier in females than in males [12]. Approximately 50% of patients diagnosed with uveal melanoma will die as a result of hematogenous spread of metastases, often to the liver [13, 14]. Unfortunately, there is usually significant tumor burden from metastases to the liver by the time liver function tests (LFTs) or imaging studies show abnormalities [15]. Following detection of metastatic disease, the median survival time is extremely poor, ranging from 2 months to about 1 year [16–18]. Currently there are no standard of care treatments for UM; however several therapies are under investigation in multicenter clinical trials.

Early diagnosis of UM is important because it not only allows for appropriate intervention to reduce the risk of metastasis but also allots patients more time to make important life decisions and manage their medical care.

Several key clinical and histopathologic observations are helpful for determining the prognosis of UM. Poor prognosis is correlated with features such as a larger tumor basal diameter, ciliary involvement, extrascleral extension, an epithelioid cell type, greater mean diameter of the ten largest nucleoli, presence of mitotic figures, presence of lymphocytic infiltrates, and abnormal microcirculation architecture [19–22].

Clinical High-Risk Features

Older Age

Age is significantly correlated with incidence of UM, with the disease more commonly seen in older adults, but rare in children [9]. For prognostication, it is reported to be a valuable and significant factor but is also purported by others to bear no significance in determining outcome from diagnosis of UM [14, 19, 23, 24]. The actual impact of age on prognosis of patients with UM is unclear because older patients often have other comorbidities or may have had UM for longer—leading to greater chance of other high-risk features including larger tumor diameter, extraocular extension, or metastasis [25].

Largest Tumor Diameter

Numerous studies cite that the largest basal tumor diameter (LTD) is the best predictor of metastatic disease [13, 18, 26–28]. It is the most widely used clinical factor for prognostication and correlates well with extraocular spread and likelihood of recurrence [29, 30]. In 2009, Damato et al. investigated the significance of LTD in posterior uveal melanoma (involving the ciliary body or choroid) along with histological and cytogenetic predictors of mortality and found that metastatic death correlated with LTD [25]. Stratifying risk factors by largest basal tumor diameter, it was found that predictors of metastatic death were most prevalent in tumors with a greater LTD [25]. Tumor thickness is also a significant prognostic factor on morbidity and mortality, as well as a predictive factor for metastasis. Each millimeter increase in thickness imparts a 1.06 hazard ratio, except in melanomas less than 1 mm in thickness in the iris or less than 2 mm in thickness in the ciliary body and choroid, likely because these thinner melanomas include high-risk diffuse melanomas [31].

Ciliary Body Involvement

UM that involve the ciliary body lead to greater mortality rates than those that do not involve the ciliary body. Its location makes diagnosis more difficult as it is hidden by the iris and unlikely to cause visual symptoms until it has grown to considerable size. These also include large choroid melanomas that reach the ciliary body. Ultimately, diagnosis of UM involving the ciliary body often occurs when it has grown large. The route for extraocular spread of melanoma from the ciliary body is the aqueous channel. A multivariate survival analysis [32] for choroidal-ciliary body melanomas found that there was a significant association between involvement of the ciliary body and mortality rates. They found that UM with ciliary body involvement was significantly more likely to be of a mixed cell type, with larger nucleoli, and have a larger tumor base, all factors that are associated with higher mortality.

Extraocular Extension

Several possible routes for extraocular extension (EOE) of UM include the aqueous drainage channels of Schlemm's canal, the anterior and posterior ciliary arteries, the four vortex veins, the long and short ciliary nerves, the optic nerve, and finally, direct scleral perforation [33]. The size of extraocular tumor has been associated with increased mortality and orbital recurrence [33, 34]. A review of the histopathologic and cytogenetic analysis of patients with UM who were treated by enucleation found that EOE was present in 14.6% of patients and was strongly correlated with large basal tumor diameter, anterior tumor extension/angle involvement, epithelioid cellularity, and closed connective tissue loops [35]. These findings indicate that the route of EOE is dependent on the UM location and that extraocular spread is an indicator of greater malignancy and tumor size.

Diffuse Pattern

A diffuse pattern of UM is rare and represents only about 5% of posterior uveal melanomas (ciliary body and choroidal). These lesions are typically minimally elevated, with a predominantly horizontal growth pattern and a large basal tumor diameter. Diffuse-type tumors have been associated with high-risk features such as epithelioid cell type and EOE and inevitably lead to a poor prognosis [36, 37]. The poor prognosis is also due to the difficulty in diagnosing these lesions clinically, as they are frequently misdiagnosed or diagnosed late. Therefore, a correct diagnosis is crucial for improving the chance of survival for the patient. Key clinical signs in diagnosing diffuse uveal melanoma are tumor thickness ≥ 2 mm, location near the optic disc, the presence of lipofuscin or subretinal fluid, or complaints of symptoms such as pain or blurring of vision [38].

Ring Melanoma

This is a very rare variant of UM in which the tumor is often found with circumferential growth around the eye. It involves the ciliary body and is usually quite advanced at the time of diagnosis, usually done by gonioscopy or ultrasound biomicroscopy [9, 39]. Reasons for advanced disease at diagnosis are similar as with ciliary body UM. Patients have few symptoms, but when they do, the most frequent symptom is blurry vision, which is improved by refractive lenses and dismissed. The blurry vision is likely due to the compressive effects of the tumor subluxating the lens. Other symptoms of ring melanoma include increased or decreased intraocular pressure, retinal or choroidal detachments and choroidal effusions, episcleral sentinel vessels, shallowing of the anterior chamber, and lens changes, all of which can add confusion to the clinical picture and complicate diagnosis [40–42].

Optic Nerve Involvement

The rate of infiltration of the optic nerve by UM has been quoted as between 0.6% and 5% of cases of UM. There is an association with juxtapapillary location, non-spindle cell type, high intraocular pressure, and blindness [43–45]. Recently, large basal tumor diameter was found to be a highly statistically significant risk factor for optic nerve spread, and a weaker correlation was found with mitotic rate [30]. However optic nerve invasion was not found to be a significant factor in survival when it was included in a multivariate analysis [27].

Histological High-Risk Features

Cell Type

Four cell types in uveal melanoma are categorized and differentiated—spindle cell nevus, spindle cell melanoma (consisting of either spindle A or B cells), epithelioid cell melanoma, and mixed-cell melanoma [46]. Spindle cells are typically well-differentiated melanocytes, most often seen in small tumors in the early stages of disease. These cells have long, oval-shaped nuclei, which may contain nucleoli, and are highly cohesive and fusiform in shape. Epithelioid cells on the other hand are poorly differentiated melanocytes. They appear as large, polyhedral cells with abundant cytoplasm and large round-to-oval nuclei with prominent nucleoli and can occasionally appear as multinucleated cells. They lack cohesion and are typically spaced far apart in the tumor architecture. Epithelioid cells have a more pleomorphic appearance than spindle cells do and are seen more frequently in large tumors, indicating the more aggressive nature of the tumor.

Mixed-cell melanomas are composed of both spindle and epithelioid cell types. The importance of cell type in a melanoma has been strongly linked to tumor growth and mortality rates. It was found that independent of tumor size, cell type was a significant prognostic indicator for mortality. The mortality rates for spindle cell type vs. epithelioid cell type in small tumors (<10 mm) were 6.5% and 47%, respectively, and for larger tumors, the mortality rates were 18% and 64%, respectively [47]. Epithelioid cell type has also been found to be a predictor for recurrence following local transscleral resection of UM [48].

Mean Diameter of the Ten Largest Nucleoli

The mean diameter of the ten largest nucleoli (MLN) is a value derived by measuring the largest diameter of the nucleoli of tumor cells on cross section cut from an

FFPE tumor tissue sample. The method itself requires an experienced observer, but when considering the variability in the methods used to obtain this value, it is apparent that there may be considerable inter-observer variability. Studies report discordant results with respect to the significance of MLN on prognostic determination, which may be due to varying protocols [28, 35, 49]. It seems that with the assistance of immunostaining, the accuracy of MLN determination has improved its significance in Cox analyses and hence its prognostic potential.

High Mitotic Rate

The presence of mitotic figures indicates proliferative activity in tissues. The conventional way to establish the degree of proliferative activity is to calculate the mitotic count. One [50] tried a new technique—the use of phospho-histone H3 (PHH3), an antibody marker used for mitotic counting in other types of tumors [51, 52]. The greater counts found by using PHH3 staining aided in drawing a significant correlation between mitotic count and the presence of extracellular matrix loops. Both markers showed a similar correlation with metastatic death, concluding that a high mitotic count was associated with an increased risk of metastasis.

Microcirculation

Uveal melanomas disseminate hematogenously, and so angiogenesis plays a key role in the biology of UM and metastasis [53]. There are two aspects of angiogenesis in tumor biology that promote tumorigenicity— remodeling of the vascular bed and production of new blood vessels [54]. The microcirculation patterns found in UM tumors have been described: closed vascular loops, incomplete vascular loops (arcs) with and without branching, microvascular networks composed of back-to-back loops, PAS-positive parallel vascular channels with and without cross-linking, incorporation of normal vessels into the tumor, and focal avascular zones [55]. In ciliary body and choroidal nevi, only four vascular patterns have been observed: normal vessels, straight vessels, parallel vessels without cross-linking, and avascular zones [56]. Interestingly, the melanomas that had nevus-like vascular patterns tended to be both smaller and located posterior to the equator than melanomas, which exhibited vascular patterns not found in choroidal nevi. In addition, the mortality rate associated with melanomas that lacked a nevus-like microcirculation was more than double that for melanomas with a nevus-like vascular pattern. In conclusion, there are three types of melanocytic uveal lesions: benign nevi with no capacity for metastasis, melanomas with a nevus-like microcirculation that have a limited capacity for metastasis associated with better prognosis and survival times, and melanomas with aggressive vascular patterns that are strongly associated with metastasis and poorer prognosis. It has been found that at 10 years post-diagnosis, survival was significantly better in patients who did not have tumors with loops, networks, or parallel vessels with cross-linking patterns [55]. The presence of networks was associated with epithelioid cell type and the absence of this cell type was associated with avascular zones [21]. The association between loops or networks and death from metastatic disease has been confirmed by several studies [22, 28, 49].

Pigmentation

Uveal melanomas exhibit varying colors, ranging from an amelanotic yellow-white to dark brown, with approximately 25% of all UM being amelanotic. In addition to the pigmentation provided by melanin in the cells, the color of the tumors can vary according to the presence of blood vessels, lipofuscin, and subretinal fluid on the surface of the tumor. On histological examination, the true degree of pigmentation of the tumor becomes apparent, and it is this factor used in prognostication. The Collaborative Ocular Melanoma Study (COMS) found an association between tumor size, cell type, and degree of pigmentation: larger tumors and an epithelioid cell type were associated with heavy pigmentation [57]. Interestingly, increasing pigmentation, larger size, and epithelioid cell type were all associated with greater number of macrophages, which in turn were associated significantly with necrosis. Heavy pigmentation has been associated with a poor prognosis [18, 58]. The degree of pigmentation in large tumors influenced the prognostic outcome if the tumor ruptured through Bruch's membrane, and mortality increased from 19% for amelanotic lesions to 65% for heavily pigmented tumors [59].

Inflammation

Inflammation is characterized by the presence of a lymphocytic infiltrate and increased expression of HLA antigens, and it is an indicator of poor prognosis in UM [60]. Since the eye is an immune privileged site, an immune response in the eye suggests extrascleral spread of UM through hematogenous routes. Hence, this will only be found in uveal melanomas that have already metastasized.

Immunohistochemical Markers

The immunohistochemical stains that have been most used in prognostic testing of uveal melanoma are HMB-45, S100, Ki-67, and Melan-A.

HMB-45 is a monoclonal antibody used as an immunohistochemical marker that is highly specific and sensitive (>90%) for cutaneous malignant [61–63]. In primary UM, HMB-45 has been shown to detect 99% of lesions, with the strongest expression of the marker at the invasive edge [64]. Overall, HMB-45 was found to be more specific and sensitive than both S100 and neuron-specific enolase in detecting uveal melanocytic tumors [65, 66].

S100 is a protein family of EF-hand calcium-binding proteins [67] whose presence is used in distinguishing between a metastatic carcinoma and a melanocytic tumor [68]. It has been found to be a sensitive marker, staining >90% of primary UM [65, 69]. However, S100 has low specificity, being expressed in many nonmelanocytic tumors, and its expression can be affected using routine FFPE tissue samples, giving false-negative results [68].

Ki-67 is a nuclear protein associated with cell proliferation rate. It has been used to detect differences in rates of cell proliferation between UM that have been irradiated and those that have not had radiation treatment [70, 71]. In 23 cases, 8 Gy irradiation was given 2 days before enucleation. Nonirradiated melanomas had a significantly higher proliferation rate as defined by staining with monoclonal antibody for Ki-67 as compared with irradiated tumors. Since a high proliferation rate of tumor cells is associated with metastasis and mortality, strong expression of Ki-67 in UM is likely an indicator of a worse prognosis. The expression of Ki-67 has also been shown to be associated with the formation of microvascular networks [72].

Melan-A is a product of the MART-1 gene and is a melanocytic differentiation antigen protein that in cutaneous melanoma has been found to be more sensitive than HMB-45 and has a higher specificity for melanocytic lesions, making it useful in diagnostic antibody panels [73]. A study that compared Melan-A with HMB-45 and S100 in ocular melanomas found that Melan-A had a higher sensitivity (100%) than HMB-45 (55%) in iris melanomas and a similar sensitivity to HMB-45 in choroidal melanomas [74].

Molecular Pathology

Intense efforts have been made over the past decades to understand the molecular genetics involved in the development and the progression of UM. Some early genetic events cause disruption of the cell cycle and apoptotic control in uveal melanocytes, and then additional disruptions lead to their malignant transformation and metastatic potential.

Cancer develops as an uncontrolled clonal proliferation of cells and acquires most or all the six hallmarks of neoplasia including (1) insensitivity to anti-growth signals, (2) self-sufficiency from growth signals, (3) avoid apoptosis, (4) limitless replicative potential, (5) sustained angiogenesis, and (6) tissue invasion and metastasis. In understanding the development of UM, it is also important to take note of the development from embryogenesis. Neural crest cells develop into nonpigmented melanoblasts that bypass natural tissue barriers and basement membranes during migration in embryogenesis. The melanoblasts mature into melanocytes within the uvea and/or give rise to melanocytic stem cells. It is hypothesized that various genetic and epigenetic alterations occur throughout the "melanoblast-melanocyte-nevus-UM" pathway, increasing the chance of malignant transformation and propensity to spread. The events include inactivating mutations or deletions of tumor (and metastasis) suppressor genes, mutation or amplification of proto-oncogenes, and larger chromosomal aberrations. It has been proposed that there are two pathways of genetic development in UM that split at an early stage: (1) class 1 gene expression profile with disomy 3 and chromosome 6p gain and (2) class 2 gene expression profile with monosomy 3—associated with a high metastatic propensity [75–78]. Later genetic events in UM development include increasing aneuploidy and chromosome 8 alterations (gains in 8q and loss of 8p).

Molecular Pathway Defects in Primary UM

In most UM, the retinoblastoma (Rb) and p53 pathways are functionally inhibited. The Rb protein is constitutively hyperphosphorylated, probably because of cyclin D1 overexpression. Increased cyclin D1 protein expression has been associated with larger tumor basal diameter, epithelioid cell type, and poor prognosis [79]. The p53 pathway is inhibited as a consequence of MDM2 overexpression, which is common in UM and associated with a poor outcome [79, 80]. PTEN inactivation also occurs and is associated with increased aneuploidy and decreased survival in UM [81, 82].

Pathways promoting growth and proliferation such as PI3K/AKT and MAPK/ERK are constitutively activated in most UM, producing inappropriate autonomous proliferation of neoplastic cells [83, 84]. The constitutive activation of the MAPK pathway in most UM suggests the presence of upstream activating mutations [85–87].

The GNAQ protein is part of the G protein subunit alpha family, which also comprises GNA11, GNA14, and GNA15/16. The mutation in GNAQ is somatically acquired, arising almost exclusively in exon 5 at codon 209, resulting in a substitution from glutamine to one of at least five known variants. Over 80% of UM were found to have GNAQ or GNA11 mutations affecting either Q209 or R183 in a mutually exclusive pattern [88]. GNAQ and GNA11 mutations are found in both uveal nevi and most UM regardless of their tumor stage, chromosomal constellation, or other predictors, suggesting that these mutations occur early in the molecular pathogenesis of UM [89].

Chromosomal Alterations in Primary UM

It has been well established for over 20 years that UM is characterized by specific chromosomal alterations distinct from cutaneous melanomas. The most unique abnormality in UM is the complete or partial loss of chromosome 3. Other common genetic abnormalities include loss on 1p, 6q, 8, and 9p, as well as gain on 1q, 6p, and 8q. Chromosome 8 gains and loss of chromosome 1 are significantly correlated with reduced survival rate [90–92]. Both chromosome 3 loss and polysomy 8q (especially when these alterations coexist) are associated with poor prognostic factors, including increasing tumor basal diameter, ciliary body involvement, presence of epithelioid cells, high mitotic count, and closed connective tissue loops [9, 90].

Conversely, gains in chromosome 6p correlate with a good prognosis, suggesting a functionally protective effect from this alteration.

Molecular Techniques Used for Prognostication in Primary UM

The most used tests are FISH, MLPA, MSA, SNP array (aSNP), and a PCR-based 12-gene assay based on gene expression profiling (GEP). GEP divides UM into two "classes" based on an mRNA expression signature [93]: class 1 and class 2. Class 1 UM often shows 6p and 8q gain and is associated with a better prognosis [75]. Class 2 UM is characterized by more aneuploidy with 1p loss, 3 loss, 8p loss, and 8q gain and is strongly associated with inactivating mutations of "BRCA1-associated protein 1" (BAP1), located at 3p21 [94]. The GEP-based test has received a considerable amount of publicity in the lay press, as it is claimed to be superior to all other testing methods [93, 95].

Molecular Alterations in UM Metastases

Aberrations of several genes and signaling pathways appear to promote dissemination of UM cells. The most convincing metastasis-regulatory gene in UM is BAP1, identified by exome sequencing [94]. The BAP1 gene encodes a deubiquitinating enzyme that binds to BRCA1 and BARD1 to form a heterodimeric tumor suppressor complex [96]. Germline BAP1 mutations have been found in families with a high risk for hereditary cancers such as mesothelioma and lung, breast, and renal cell carcinomas [97–101]. This has been described as a novel "BAP1 cancer syndrome" by several groups [98–102].

Studies using FISH to examine UM metastases demonstrated that these disseminated tumor cells are characterized by chromosome 3 loss and 8q gain [103, 104]. The metastatic process is multistepped and complex and depends on numerous alterations occurring both within the tumor and its microenvironment, and these factors may determine the location of metastases. Some potential therapies targeting these variations include inhibitors of the MAPK/MEK signaling pathway, PI3K/AKT pathway at the level of AKT, mTOR, mTOR blockade combined with an IGF-1R antibody, tyrosine kinases, c-Met pathway, CXCR4, and histone deacetylase [105]. Uveal melanoma is not characterized by BRAF or NRAS mutations, so targeted therapy for cutaneous melanoma cannot be readily applied for uveal melanoma [106].

The identification of the altered genetic pathways associated with UM oncogenesis and particularly those with metastasis is still in its preliminary stages. Characteristic copy number alterations and DNA expression profiles have been identified in UM, which are strongly correlated with prognosis. The rapidly developing field of molecular genetics will shed further light on key signaling pathways involved in UM oncogenesis and progression, opening the way for target-based therapies.

Scope of Prognostication

It is widely stated that patients with UM have a 50% chance of dying from their disease. However, it is important to note that this is a summary statistic and the prognoses for individual patients vary, with some very much better or considerably worse than the average [107]. Most cancer prognostication is based on the TNM (tumor, node, and metastasis) staging system of the American Joint Committee on Cancer (AJCC) and the Union for International Cancer Control (UICC). While the TNM staging manual helps to assess general tumor characteristics and spread, it does not yet advise on using all clinical and laboratory tumor data. However, improvements are being made to the TNM system so that it uses all available data. Progress in prognostication would be accelerated by multicenter collaboration, which should become as feasible as biopsy, histological grading as genetic typing becomes more widespread. There is scope for multicenter studies to determine whether methods used in one unit are reliable elsewhere and to compare rival techniques and strategies [107].

The accuracy of prognostication is enhanced by multivariate analysis of clinical, histological, and genetic data. Patients with a "low-risk" uveal melanoma are more likely to enjoy a good quality of life if they informed about their excellent prognosis. Patients with a high risk of metastatic disease tend to develop coping mechanisms when told of their prognosis, so that their quality of life is far better than one might expect. Improved identification of "high-risk" patients has led to targeted screening for metastatic disease and better opportunities for clinical trials evaluating different treatments for metastatic disease. More accurate prognostication also enhances prospects for randomized trials evaluating systemic adjuvant therapy as well as basic science research. The prognostic methods that have been developed for ocular oncology should be widely applicable, not only in ophthalmology and oncology but also in other fields of medicine [107].

Treatment Modalities

Treatment of primary UM includes enucleation or radiotherapy (either plaque brachytherapy or proton radiotherapy), and the decision is guided by the size and location of the tumor, presence of extraocular extension, vision, and patient preference [106]. Plaque and proton beam radiotherapy are used for small to medium ciliary body or choroidal melanomas, while enucleation is the preferred option for large posterior uveal melanomas with poor vision at presentation [9]. Both treatment modalities lead to similar survival and metastasis rates, but radiotherapy has the advantage of a better cosmetic result and the possibility to preserve vision [106]. Small choroidal melanomas can also be treated with transpupillary thermotherapy or, if it is amelanotic, photodynamic therapy [9]. If the tumor exhibits extraocular extension, orbital exenteration is likely the best choice [9].

Treatment of metastatic disease is much less effective, and the value of screening and treatment is controversial [108, 109]. Up to 50% of patients will develop systemic metastasis and 90% of these patients will have metastasis to the liver [110]. If metastatic disease is diagnosed early, the patient is more likely to benefit from liver-directed therapy [106]. Some treatment modalities are designed to control tumor progression in the liver, including surgical resection, hepatic arterial chemotherapy, transarterial chemoembolization (TACE), or isolated hepatic perfusion with melphalan [106, 110]. Since there is no standard of care for patients with metastatic uveal melanoma, several clinical trials are testing the efficacy of the PKC inhibitors AEB071 and LXS196, MEK inhibitors MEK162 and selumetinib, and immune checkpoint inhibitors like ipilimumab [106]. The best results are among patients with solitary hepatic metastases and have received surgery, ablative procedures, or isolated hepatic perfusion with melphalan [106]. The use of these local therapies led to patients having the best 1-year survival rates at 82.1%, compared to 49% in those receiving systemic therapy or 27.5% in those receiving only supportive care [106]. The use of immune checkpoint inhibitors for metastatic UM is still being investigated, but current evidence suggest that it has limited efficacy [106, 111].

References

1. Demato B, Coupland S. Differences in uveal melanomas between men and women from the British Isles. Eye (Lond). 2012;26(2):292–9.
2. Egan K, Seddon J, Glynn R, Gragoudas E, Albert D. Epidemiologic aspects of uveal melanoma. Surv Ophthalmol. 1988;32(4):239–51.
3. Gallagher RP, Elwood JM, Rootman J, Spinelli JJ, Hill GB, Threlfall WJ, et al. Risk factors for ocular melanoma: Western Canada Melanoma Study. J Natl Cancer Inst. 1985;74(4):775–8.
4. Seddon J, Gragoudas E, Egan K, Albert D, Blitzer P, Glynn R. Host factors, UV radiation, and risk of uveal melanoma. A case-control study. Arch Ophthalmol. 1990;108(9):1274–80.
5. Singh A, Bergman L, Seregard S. Uveal melanoma: epidemiologic aspects. Ophthalmol Clin N Am. 2005;18(1):75–84.
6. Hu D, Yu G, McCormick S, Finger P. Population-based incidence of uveal melanoma in various races and ethnic groups. Am J Ophthalmol. 2005;140(4):612–7.
7. Margo C, Mulla Z, Billiris K. Incidence of surgically treated uveal melanoma by race and ethnicity. Ophthalmology. 1998;105(6):1087–90.
8. Singh A, Topham A. Incidence of uveal melanoma in the United States: 1973-1997. Ophthalmology. 2003;110(5):956–61.
9. Kaliki S, Shields CL. Uveal melanoma: relatively rare but deadly cancer. Eye. 2017;31(2):241–57.
10. Singh A, Turell M, Topham A. Uveal melanoma: trends in incidence, treatment, and survival. Ophthalmology. 2011;118(9):1881–5.
11. van Hees CLM, Bergman W, de Boer A, Jager MJ, Bleeker JC, Kakebeeke HM, et al. Are atypical nevi a risk factor for uveal melanoma? A case-control study. J Invest Dermatol. 1994;103(2):202–5.
12. Bergman L, Seregard S, Bilsson B, Ringborg U, Lundell G, Ragnarsson-Olding B. Incidence of uveal melanoma in Sweden from 1960 to 1998. Invest Ophthalmol Vis Sci. 2002;43(8):2579–83.
13. Kujala E, Mäkitie T, Kivelä T. Very long-term prognosis of patients with malignant uveal melanoma. Invest Ophthalmol Vis Sci. 2003;44(11):4651–9.
14. Stegan S, Erik K. Prognostic indicators following enucleation for posterior uveal melanoma. Acta Ophthalmol. 1995;73(4):340–4.

15. Kaiserman I, Amer R, Pe'er J. Liver function tests in metastatic uveal melanoma. Am J Ophthalmol. 2004;137(2):236–43.
16. Bedikian AY. Metastatic Uveal melanoma therapy. Int Ophthalmol Clin. 2006;46(1):151–66.
17. Kath R, Hayungs J, Bornfeld N, Sauerwein W, Höffken K, Seeber S. Prognosis and treatment of disseminated uveal melanoma. Cancer. 1993;72(7):2219–23.
18. Seddonn J, Albert D, Lavin P, Robinson N. A prognostic factor study of disease-free interval and survival following enucleation for uveal melanoma. Arch Ophthalmol. 1983;101(1):1894–9.
19. Augsburger J, Gamel J. Clinical prognostic factors in patients with posterior uveal malignant melanoma. Cancer. 1990;66(7):1596–600.
20. De Cruz P, Specht C, McLean I. Lymphocytic infiltration in uveal malignant melanoma. Cancer. 1990;65(1):112–5.
21. Folberg R, Re'er J, Gruman WR, Jeng G, Montague P, et al. The morphologic characteristics of tumor blood vessels as a marker of tumor progression in primary human uveal melanoma: a matched case-control study. Hum Pathol. 1992;23(11):1298–305.
22. Mäkitie T, Summanen P, Tarkkanen A, Kivelä T. Microvascular loops and networks as prognostic indicators in choroidal and ciliary body melanomas. J Natl Cancer Inst. 1999;91(4):359–67.
23. Survival from uveal melanoma in England and Wales 1986 to 2001. Ophthalmic Epidemiol. 2007;14(1):3–8.
24. Diener-West M, Earle J, Fine S, Hawkins B, Moy C, Reynolds S, et al. The COMS randomized trial of iodine 125 brachytherapy for choroidal melanoma, II: characteristics of patients enrolled and not enrolled. COMS report no. 17. Arch Ophthalmol. 2001;119(7):951–65.
25. Damato B, Coupland SE. A reappraisal of the significance of largest basal diameter of posterior uveal melanoma. Eye. 2009;23(12):2152–62.
26. Diener-West M, Reynolds S, Agugliaro D, Caldwell R, Cumming K, Earle J, et al. Development of metastatic disease after enrollment in the COMS trials for treatment of choroidal melanoma: collaborative ocular melanoma study group report no. 26. Arch Ophthalmol. 2005;123(12):1639–43.
27. Isager P, Ehlers N, Overgaard J. Prognostic factors for survival after enucleation for choroidal and ciliary body melanomas. Acta Ophthalmol Scand. 2004;82(5):517–25.
28. McLean I, Keefe K, Burnier M. Uveal melanoma. Comparison of the prognostic value of fibrovascular loops, mean of the ten largest nucleoli, cell type, and tumor size. Ophthalmology. 1997;104(5):777–80.
29. Bellmann C, Lumbroso-Le Rouic L, Levy C, Plancher C, Dendale R, Sastre-Garau X, et al. Uveal melanoma: management and outcome of patients with extraocular spread. Br J Ophthalmol. 2009;94(5):569–74.
30. Coupland S, Campbell I, Damato B. Routes of extraocular extension of uveal melanoma: risk factors and influence on survival probability. Ophthalmology. 2008;115(10):1778–85.
31. Shields CL, Furuta M, Thangappan A, Nagori S, Mashayekhi A, Lally DR, et al. Metastasis of uveal melanoma millimeter-by-millimeter in 8033 consecutive eyes. Arch Ophthalmol. 2009;127(8):989–98.
32. McLean I, Ainbinder D, Gamel J, McCurdy J, Choroidal-ciliary body melanoma. A multivariate survival analysis of tumor location. Ophthalmology. 1995;102(7):1060–4.
33. Pach J, Robertson D, Taney B, Martin J, Cambell R, O'Brien P. Prognostic factors in choroidal and ciliary body melanomas with extrascleral extension. Am J Ophthalmol. 1986;101(3):325–31.
34. Affeldt JC, Minckler DS, Azen SP, Yeh L. Prognosis in Uveal melanoma with extrascleral extension. Arch Ophthalmol. 1980;98(11):1975–9.
35. Swthi K, Carol LS, Jerry AS. Uveal melanoma: estimating prognosis. Indian J Ophthalmol. 2015;63(2):93–102.
36. Font RL, Spaulding AG, Zimmerman LE. Diffuse malignant melanoma of the uveal tract: a clinicopathologic report of 54 cases. Trans Am Acad Ophthalmol Otolaryngol. 1968;72(6):877–95.

References

37. Reese A, Howard G. Flat uveal melanomas. Am J Ophthalmol. 1967;64(6):1021–8.
38. Shields C, Shields J, Kiratli H, De Potter P, Cater J. Risk factors for growth and metastasis of small choroidal melanocytic lesions. Ophthalmology. 1995;102(9):1351–61.
39. Wilkinson CP. Book reviews: atlas of intraocular tumors. Retina. 1999;19(6):580.
40. Chaudhry I, Moster M, Augsburger J. Iris ring melanoma masquerading as pigmentary glaucoma. Arch Ophthalmol. 1997;115(11):1480–1.
41. Diekstall F, Demeler U. Therapy-resistant increase in ocular pressure—a rare differential diagnosis: ring melanoma. Fortschr Ophthalmol. 1988;85(1):98–100.
42. Vásquez LM, Pavlin CJ, McGowan H, Simpson ER. Ring melanoma of the ciliary body: clinical and ultrasound biomicroscopic characteristics. Can J Ophthalmol. 2008;43(2):229–33.
43. Christmas N, Mead M, Richardson E, Albert D. Secondary optic nerve tumors. Surv Ophthalmol. 1991;36(3):196–206.
44. Lindegaard J, Heegaard S, Prause J. Histopathologically verified non-vascular optic nerve lesions in Denmark 1940-99. Acta Ophthalmol Scand. 2002;80(1):32–7.
45. Shammas H, Blodi F. Peripapillary choroidal melanomas. Extension along the optic nerve and its sheaths. Arch Ophthalmol. 1978;96(3):440–5.
46. McLean I, Foster W, Zimmerman L, Gamel J. Modifications of Callender's classification of uveal melanoma at the Armed Forces Institute of Pathology. Am J Ophthalmol. 1983;96(4):502–9.
47. McLean M, Foster W, Zimmerman L. Prognostic factors in small malignant melanomas of choroid and ciliary body. Arch Ophthalmol. 1997;95(1):48–58.
48. Damato BE, Paul J, Foulds WS. Risk factors for residual and recurrent uveal melanoma after trans-scleral local resection. Br J Ophthalmol. 1996;80(2):102–8.
49. Seregard S, Spångberg B, Juul C, Oskarsson M. Prognostic accuracy of the mean of the largest nucleoli, vascular patterns, and PC-10 in posterior uveal melanoma. Ophthalmology. 1998;105(3):485–91.
50. Angi M, Damato B, Kalirai H, Dodson A, Taktak A, Coupland S. Immunohistochemical assessment of mitotic count in uveal melanoma. Acta Ophthalmol. 2011;89(2):155–60.
51. Tapia C, Kutzner H, Mentzel T, Savic S, Baumhoer D, Glatz K. Two mitosis-specific antibodies, MPM-2 and phospho-histone H3 (Ser28), allow rapid and precise determination of mitotic activity. Am J Surg Pathol. 2006;30(1):83–9.
52. Hale CS, Qian M, Ma MW, Scanlon P, Berman RS, Shapiro RL, et al. Mitotic rate in melanoma: prognostic value of immunostaining and computer-assisted image analysis. Am J Surg Pathol. 2013;37(6):882–9.
53. Folberg R, Mehaffey M, Gardner L, Meyer M, Rummelt V, Pe'er J. The microcirculation of choroidal and ciliary body melanomas. Eye (Lond). 1997;11(part 2):227–38.
54. Vernon R, Sage E. Between molecules and morphology. Extracellular matrix and creation of vascular form. Am J Pathol. 1995;174(4):873–83.
55. Folberg R, Rummelt V, Parys-Van Ginderdeuren R, Hwang T, Woolson R, Pe'er J, et al. The prognostic value of tumor blood vessel morphology in primary uveal melanoma. Ophthalmology. 1993;100(9):1389–98.
56. Rummelt V, Folberg R, Rummelt C, Gruman L, Hwang T, Woolson R, et al. Microcirculation architecture of melanocytic nevi and malignant melanomas of the ciliary body and choroid. A comparative histopathologic and ultrastructural study. Ophthalmology. 1994;101(4):718–27.
57. Histopathologic characteristics of uveal melanomas in eyes enucleated from the Collaborative Ocular Melanoma Study. COMS report no. 6. Am J Ophthalmol. 1998;125(6):745–66.
58. McLean I, Saraiva V, Burnier M. Pathological and prognostic features of uveal melanomas. Can J Ophthalmol. 2004;39(4):343–50.
59. Shammas HF, Blodi FC. Prognostic factors in choroidal and ciliary body melanomas. Arch Ophthalmol. 1977;95(1):63–9.
60. Inflammatory cytokines in eyes with uveal melanoma and relation with macrophage infiltration. Invest Ophthalmol Vis Sci. 2010;51(11):5445–51.

61. Gown AM, Vogel AM, Hoak D, Gough F, McNutt MA. Monoclonal antibodies specific for melanocytic tumors distinguish subpopulations of melanocytes. Am J Pathol. 1986;123(2):195–203.
62. Ordóñez NG, Xiaolong J, Hickey RC. Comparison of HMB-45 monoclonal antibody and S-100 protein in the immunohistochemical diagnosis of melanoma. Am J Clin Pathol. 1988;90(4):385–90.
63. Wick MR, Swanson PE, Rocamora A. Recognition of malignant melanoma by monoclonal antibody HMB-45. An immunohistochemical study of 200 paraffin-embedded cutaneous tumors. J Cutan Pathol. 1988;15(4):201–7.
64. Steuhl K-P, Rohrbach JM, Knorr M, Thiel H-J. Significance, specificity, and ultrastructural localization of HMB-45 antigen in pigmented ocular tumors. Ophthalmology. 1993;100(2):208–15.
65. Burnier MN, McLean IW, Gamel JW. Immunohistochemical evaluation of uveal melanocytic tumors. Expression of HMB-45, S-100 protein, and neuron-specific enolase. Cancer. 1991;68(4):809–14.
66. Luyten GPM, Mooy CM, Post J, Jensen OA, Luider TM, de Jong PTVM. Metastatic uveal melanoma: a morphologic and immunohistochemical analysis. Cancer. 1996;78(9):1967–71.
67. Schäfer BW, Heizmann CW. The S100 family of EF-hand calcium-binding proteins: functions and pathology. Trends Biochem Sci. 1996;21(4):134–40.
68. Cochran AJ, Holland GN, Wen DR, Herschman HR, Lee WR, Foos RY, et al. Detection of cytoplasmic S-100 protein in primary and metastatic intraocular melanomas. Invest Ophthalmol Vis Sci. 1983;24(8):1153–5.
69. Cochran AJ, Lu H-F, Li P-X, Saxton R, Wen D-R. S-100 protein remains a practical marker for melanocytic and other tumours. Melanoma Res. 1993;3(5):325–30.
70. Mooy CM, De Jong PTVM, Van Der Kwast TH, Mulder PGH, Jager MJ, Ruiter DJ. Ki-67 immunostaining in uveal melanoma. Ophthalmology. 1990;97(10):1275–80.
71. Schilling H, Sehu KW, Lee WR. A histologic study (including DNA quantification and Ki-67 labeling index) in uveal melanomas after brachytherapy with ruthenium plaques. Invest Ophthalmol Vis Sci. 1997;38(10):2081–92.
72. Chowers I. Comparison of microcirculation patterns and MIB-1 immunoreactivity in iris and posterior uveal melanoma. Ophthalmology. 2001;108(2):367–71.
73. Blessing S, Grant. Comparison of immunohistochemical staining of the novel antibody melan-A with S100 protein and HMB-45 in malignant melanoma and melanoma variants. Histopathology. 1998;32(2):139–46.
74. Heegaard S, Jensen OA, Prause JU. Immunohistochemical diagnosis of malignant melanoma of the conjunctiva and uvea: comparison of the novel antibody against melan-a with S100 protein and HMB-45. Melanoma Res. 2000;10(4):350–4.
75. Harbour JW. The genetics of uveal melanoma: an emerging framework for targeted therapy. Pigment Cell Melanoma Res. 2012;25(2):171–81.
76. Höglund M, Gisselsson D, Hansen GB, White VA, Säll T, Mitelman F, et al. Dissecting karyotypic patterns in malignant melanomas: temporal clustering of losses and gains in melanoma karyotypic evolution. Int J Cancer. 2003;108(1):57–65.
77. Parrella P, Sidransky D, Merbs SL. Allelotype of posterior uveal melanoma: implications for a bifurcated tumor progression pathway. Cancer Res. 1999;59(13):3032–7.
78. Tschentscher F, Hüsing J, Hölter T, Kruse E, Dresen IG, Jöckel K-H, et al. Tumor classification based on gene expression profiling shows that uveal melanomas with and without monosomy 3 represent two distinct entities. Cancer Res. 2003;63(10):2578–84.
79. Coupland SE, Anastassiou G, Stang A, Schilling H, Anagnostopoulos I, Bornfeld N, et al. The prognostic value of cyclin D1, p53, and MDM2 protein expression in uveal melanoma. J Pathol. 2000;191(2):120–6.
80. Brantley MA Jr, Harbour JW. Deregulation of the Rb and p53 pathways in uveal melanoma. Am J Pathol. 2000;157(6):1795–801.

81. Abdel-Rahman MH, Yang Y, Zhou X-P, Craig EL, Davidorf FH, Eng C. High frequency of submicroscopic hemizygous deletion is a major mechanism of loss of expression of PTEN in uveal melanoma. J Clin Oncol. 2006;24(2):288–95.
82. Ehlers JP, Worley L, Onken MD, Harbour JW. Integrative genomic analysis of aneuploidy in uveal melanoma. Clin Cancer Res. 2008;14(1):115–22.
83. Babchia N, Calipel A, Mouriaux F, Faussat A-M, Mascarelli F. The PI3K/Akt and mTOR/P70S6K signaling pathways in human uveal melanoma cells: interaction with B-Raf/ERK. Invest Opthalmol Visual Sci. 2010;51(1):421.
84. Denhardt DT. Signal-transducing protein phosphorylation cascades mediated by Ras/Rho proteins in the mammalian cell: the potential for multiplex signalling. Biochem J. 1996;318(3):729–47.
85. An J, Wan H, Zhou X, Hu D-N, Wang L, Hao L, et al. A comparative transcriptomic analysis of uveal melanoma and normal uveal melanocyte. PLoS One. 2011;6(1):e16516.
86. Weber A, Hengge UR, Urbanik D, Markwart A, Mirmohammadsaegh A, Reichel MB, et al. Absence of mutations of the BRAF gene and constitutive activation of extracellular-regulated kinase in malignant melanomas of the uvea. Lab Investig. 2003;83(12):1771–6.
87. Zuidervaart W, van Nieuwpoort F, Stark M, Dijkman R, Packer L, Borgstein A-M, et al. Activation of the MAPK pathway is a common event in uveal melanomas although it rarely occurs through mutation of BRAF or RAS. Br J Cancer. 2005;92(11):2032–8.
88. Van Raamsdonk CD, Griewank KG, Crosby MB, Garrido MC, Vemula S, Wiesner T, et al. Mutations in GNA11 in uveal melanoma. New Eng J Med. 2010;363(23):2191–9.
89. Bauer J, Kilic E, Vaarwater J, Bastian BC, Garbe C, de Klein A. Oncogenic GNAQ mutations are not correlated with disease-free survival in uveal melanoma. Br J Cancer. 2009;101(5):813–5.
90. Damato B, Dopierala JA, Coupland SE. Genotypic profiling of 452 choroidal melanomas with multiplex ligation-dependent probe amplification. Clin Cancer Res. 2010;16(24):6083–92.
91. Sisley K, Rennie IG, Parsons MA, Jacques R, Hammond DW, Bell SM, et al. Abnormalities of chromosomes 3 and 8 in posterior uveal melanoma correlate with prognosis. Genes Chromosomes Cancer. 1997;19(1):22–8.
92. Damato B, Duke C, Coupland SE, Hiscott P, Smith PA, Campbell I, et al. Cytogenetics of uveal melanoma. Ophthalmology. 2007;114(10):1925–1931.e1.
93. Onken MD, Worley LA, Char DH, Augsburger JJ, Correa ZM, Nudleman E, et al. Collaborative ocular oncology group report number 1: prospective validation of a multi-gene prognostic assay in uveal melanoma. Ophthalmology. 2012;119(8):1596–603.
94. Harbour JW, Onken MD, Roberson EDO, Duan S, Cao L, Worley LA, et al. Frequent mutation of BAP1 in metastasizing uveal melanomas. Science. 2010;330(6009):1410–3.
95. Onken MD, Worley LA, Tuscan MD, Harbour JW. An accurate, clinically feasible multi-gene expression assay for predicting metastasis in Uveal melanoma. J Mol Diagn. 2010;12(4):461–8.
96. Laurent C, Valet F, Planque N, Silveri L, Maacha S, Anezo O, et al. High PTP4A3 phosphatase expression correlates with metastatic risk in uveal melanoma patients. Cancer Res. 2010;71(3):666–74.
97. Jensen DE, Proctor M, Marquis ST, Gardner HP, Ha SI, Chodosh LA, et al. BAP1: a novel ubiquitin hydrolase which binds to the BRCA1 RING finger and enhances BRCA1-mediated cell growth suppression. Oncogene. 1998;16(9):1097–112.
98. Abdel-Rahman MH, Pilarski R, Cebulla CM, Massengill JB, Christopher BN, Boru G, et al. Germline BAP1 mutation predisposes to uveal melanoma, lung adenocarcinoma, meningioma, and other cancers. J Med Genet. 2011;48(12):856–9.
99. Wiesner T, Obenauf AC, Murali R, Fried I, Griewank KG, Ulz P, et al. Germline mutations in BAP1 predispose to melanocytic tumors. Nat Genet. 2011;43(10):1018–21.
100. Testa JR, Cheung M, Pei J, Below JE, Tan Y, Sementino E, et al. Germline BAP1 mutations predispose to malignant mesothelioma. Nat Genet. 2011;43(10):1022–5.

101. Njauw C-NJ, Kim I, Piris A, Gabree M, Taylor M, Lane AM, et al. Germline BAP1 inactivation is preferentially associated with metastatic ocular melanoma and cutaneous-ocular melanoma families. PLoS One. 2012;7(4):e35295.
102. Carbone M, Ferris LK, Baumann F, Napolitano A, Lum CA, Flores EG, et al. BAP1 cancer syndrome: malignant mesothelioma, uveal and cutaneous melanoma, and MBAITs. J Transl Med [Internet]. 2012;10:1. https://doi.org/10.1186/1479-5876-10-179.
103. Singh AD, Aronow ME, Sun Y, Bebek G, Saunthararajah Y, Schoenfield LR, et al. Chromosome 3 status in Uveal melanoma: a comparison of fluorescence in situ hybridization and single-nucleotide polymorphism array. Invest Ophthalmol Vis Sci. 2012;53(7):3331.
104. Aalto Y, Eriksson L, Seregard S, Larsson O, Knuutila S. Concomitant loss of chromosome 3 and whole arm losses and gains of chromosome 1, 6, or 8 in metastasizing primary uveal melanoma. Invest Ophthalmol Vis Sci. 2001;42(2):313–7.
105. Landreville S, Agapova OA, Matatall KA, Kneass ZT, Onken MD, Lee RS, et al. Histone deacetylase inhibitors induce growth arrest and differentiation in uveal melanoma. Clin Cancer Res. 2011;18(2):408–16.
106. Jochems A, van der Kooij MK, Fiocco M, Schouwenburg MG, Aarts MJ, van Akkooi AC, et al. Metastatic uveal melanoma: treatment strategies and survival—results from the dutch melanoma treatment registry. Cancers (Basel). 2019;11:7. [Internet]. Available from: https://www.ncbi.nlm.nih.gov/pmc/articles/PMC6678641/ [cited 2020 Aug 5]
107. Damato B, Eleuteri A, Taktak AFG, Coupland SE. Estimating prognosis for survival after treatment of choroidal melanoma. Prog Retin Eye Res. 2011;30(5):285–95.
108. Augsburger JJ, Corrêa ZM, Shaikh AH. Effectiveness of treatments for metastatic melanoma. Am J Ophthalmol. 2009;148(1):119–27.
109. Kim IK. Survival in patients with presymptomatic diagnosis of metastatic uveal melanoma. Arch Ophthalmol. 2010;128(7):871.
110. Sato T. Locoregional management of hepatic metastasis from primary uveal melanoma. Semin Oncol. 2010;37(2):127–38.
111. Heppt MV, Steeb T, Schlager JG, Rosumeck S, Dressler C, Ruzicka T, et al. Immune checkpoint blockade for unresectable or metastatic uveal melanoma: a systematic review. Cancer Treat Rev. 2017;60:44–52.

Conjunctival Melanoma

Conjunctival melanoma (CoM) is rare, constituting about just 2% of all ocular malignancies and 5% of all ocular melanoma [1, 2]. CoM is the second most frequent malignant neoplasm of the conjunctiva after squamous cell carcinoma [3].

Terminology and Classification of Early Lesions

Melanosis describes melanotic pigmentation that is visible to the naked eye, which can represent freckles, nevi, neoplasia, or secondary processes like squamous cell carcinoma, ochronosis, or Addison's disease. The cause of melanosis can be hypermelanosis, which is melanin overproduction and accumulation in the cytoplasm of melanocytes or epithelial cells, or melanocytic proliferation. Melanocytic proliferations within the epithelium can be described as "primary acquired melanosis" (PAM) [4]. This was suggested to be too vague, so proposals have been made to rename it into "conjunctival melanocytic intraepithelial neoplasia (C-MIN) [4]. By assessing cytologic features of the melanocytes histologically for pleomorphism, prominent nucleoli, mitotic figures, or epithelioid cells, C-MIN can be further classified as being with or without atypia [4]. The classification of advanced C-MIN with atypia eventually blurs into conjunctival melanoma in situ.

C-MIN presents at a median age of 56 years as unilateral, unifocal, or multifocal conjunctival melanosis and is brown, flat, and irregular. This pigmentation tends to "wax and wane" with an increase or decrease in horizontal extension [5]. Furthermore, not all conjunctival melanocytic lesions are pigmented, and involvement of the cornea is possible [1, 6–8]. The prevalence of conjunctival melanocytic lesions is reported to be up to 36% in Caucasians and 4% in non-Caucasians, with a higher incidence in female patients [9].

To provide a more objective and reproducible classification, a scoring system is developed for C-MIN based on the pattern of horizontal epithelial involvement, vertical depth of melanocytic infiltration of the epithelium, degree of cellular atypia, nuclear and cellular diameter, as well as the prominence of nucleoli and mitotic figures. The C-MIN score ranges from 0 to 10, with 0 equating to "melanosis only," 1 equating to "C-MIN with mild atypia," 2–3 for "C-MIN with moderate atypia," 4 for "C-MIN with severe atypia," and a score greater than 5 for "conjunctival melanoma in situ"—meaning confluent melanocytic proliferation involving 50% of the epithelium thickness [10]. The differential diagnosis of C-MIN includes causes of hypermelanosis (i.e., freckle or complexion melanosis), secondary melanosis (i.e., from Addison's disease), pigmented squamous cell carcinoma, and subconjunctival pigmentation (i.e., congenital ocular melanocytosis) [6]. Treatment of C-MIN/PAM is aimed at preventing the development of invasive melanoma, though there is no consensus as to the best form of management. Some advocate periodic observation of small lesions [5]. Therapeutic methods include excision with adjunctive cryotherapy, with or without an amniotic-membrane graft [5, 11, 12], and topical chemotherapy with mitomycin C, 5-fluoro-uracil, and interferon alpha-2-beta [9, 13–15]. The current trend is leaning toward topical chemotherapy [14, 16].

Conjunctival melanocytic lesions without atypia rarely exhibit recurrence, whereas C-MIN with atypia recur in nearly 60% of cases after excision alone at a mean time of 2.5 years, half of which recur in the form of invasive melanoma [17].

Conjunctival Melanoma (CoM)

CoM has an incidence of 0.2–0.8 per million individuals per year in the Caucasian population, with only rare cases being reported in the non-Caucasians [1, 3, 18]. Like cutaneous melanoma, and unlike uveal melanoma, the incidence has been increasing over the past few decades, possibly due to increased environmental exposure to ultraviolet light [19]. The incidence is equal between men and women or slightly higher in men [2, 3, 18]. Up to 70% of invasive conjunctival melanomas arise from C-MIN, up to 25% from nevi, and rarely de novo [1, 2, 5, 6, 20–23]. Nevi present in childhood and that increase in size during adulthood indicates likely malignant transformation [24]. CoM is a unilateral disease that presents in adulthood at a median age of 60 years and is rare in childhood [25]. These tumors commonly arise in the perilimbal, interpalpebral, or bulbar conjunctiva, the plica semilunaris, or the caruncle [19]. CoM typically presents as an asymptomatic raised pigmented plaque, macule, or tumor of variable size [19]. Invasive conjunctival melanomas are found mostly as a singular lesion in an individual but can present as multifocal tumors in rare cases [6]. Its features can be variable, presenting as pigmented or nonpigmented; the edges can be discrete, diffuse, or mixed; and about 50% are associated with C-MIN [4]. Features to look for are large tumor size, diverse appearance, lack of mobility relative to the sclera, extension into the cornea, and presence of large feeder vessels [19].

Corneal involvement may result from tumors adjacent to the limbus, but Bowman's membrane acts as a barrier against deep invasion [1]. CoM can spread locally into the globe or orbit, to the nasolacrimal system, or into the sinuses, and then further metastasize by lymphatic or hematogenous routes [2, 10, 23]. Local tumor seeding to the adjacent lid or skin can also accidentally occur by inoculation of tissues during excision or harvesting mucous membrane for grafting using contaminated instruments [10, 26].

CoM shows invasion of atypical melanocytes from the overlying conjunctival epithelium penetrating the basement membrane into the subepithelial connective tissue (substantia propria) [6]. Histopathologic evaluation of peripheral and deep margins with respect to tumor infiltration is necessary.

The differential diagnosis includes (1) conjunctival nevi, which usually arises in childhood or adolescence, occurs most commonly in the bulbar conjunctiva and caruncle, and usually contains clear cysts; (2) squamous cell carcinoma and conjunctival squamous intra-epithelial neoplasia that are usually amelanotic, but can acquire pigmentation and resemble CoM; (3) rare lesions such as staphylomas, subconjunctival hematomas, foreign bodies, and hematic cysts; (4) epibulbar extension of uveal melanoma and melanocytoma, which may require high-frequency ultrasonography for detection [27]; and (5) metastatic cutaneous melanoma [28]. Excisional biopsy is preferred over incisional biopsy, which is dangerous because it can cause seeding if the tumor is a melanoma.

Genetic Abnormalities

Investigations of the CoM genetic pathogenesis show similarity to that of cutaneous melanoma because of frequent BRAF V600E mutations [29, 30], and an additional 18% of CoMs have NRAS mutations [24, 31]. Using multiplex ligation-dependent probe amplification (MLPA), the presence of the BRAF V600E mutation has been confirmed in 50% of primary and metastatic CoM [32]. Now all CoMs are routinely tested for the BRAF V600E mutation, which may predict responsiveness to vemurafenib should the patient develop metastatic disease [33]. Combination therapy with BRAF and MEK inhibitors dabrafenib and trametinib has shown clinical benefit, with some cases of patients exhibiting complete regression of local disease 1 year after treatment [34–37].

Primary CoM appears to have genetic alterations different from metastatic CoM. In primary tumors, CDKN1A and RUNX2 (both on 6p21.2) are amplified. Conversely, metastatic CoMs frequently show amplifications in MLH1 (3p22.1) and TIMP2 (17q25.3), while MGMT (20q26.3) and ECHS1 (10q26.3) are frequently deleted [32]. Amplification analysis by P036 assay reveals that although CDKN1A and RUNX2 are both amplified and both are at 6p21.2, there is no amplification of 6p, suggesting that these genes may play a significant role in CoM development. The CDKN1A gene produces p21, which is a cell cycle inhibitor and may either have a tumor suppressive effect such as in cutaneous melanoma or promote tumor survival by protecting from excessive DNA damage [38, 39]. Increased RUNX2 expression has been associated with enhanced motility and invasion of cells in other cancers such as cutaneous melanoma [40–42], breast cancer, and prostate cancer [43, 44].

Although CoMs are histopathologically and clinically distinct from their more common intraocular counterpart, uveal melanoma (UM), studies have investigated whether UM and CoMs share molecular genetic alterations. The frequent genetic aberrations associated with uveal melanoma patient mortality are on chromosomes 1p, 3, 6, and 8 as detected by the P027 assay [45–47]. However, the P027 assay has shown that none of these gross chromosomal abnormalities are present in primary CoMs or their metastases [48]. CoMs show gains of 1q, 3p, 7, and 17q and losses of 9q, 10, 11, and 12q (1). Specifically, metastatic CoMs show frequent amplifications of 3q, 4p, 20q, and 10q, as measured by their respective representative genes BDH, FLJ20265, ORPL1, and PAO. Unlike uveal melanomas that frequently show chromosome 3 loss, the metastatic CoM samples demonstrated frequent amplification of 3q, suggesting a different molecular genetic pathogenesis for these two ocular malignancies [2].

Staging

Clinically, CoMs are staged according to the eighth edition of TNM system developed by the AJCC and the International Union for Cancer Control (UICC) (Table 12.1).

The TNM system for conjunctival melanoma has changed radically between editions, reflecting uncertainty as to the best way of classifying this tumor [49–51]. However, the current system was shown to correlate with survival and especially with local recurrence [52–54]. In particular, T2 and T3 conjunctival melanoma had higher rates of recurrence, lymph node metastasis, distant metastasis, and mortality than stage T1 [24, 53].

No other clinical feature has been consistently associated with prognosis of primary conjunctival melanoma. This highlights the importance of radical surgery combined with adequate adjuvant therapy such as topical mitomycin or brachytherapy. Adjuvant treatment is especially important in the presence of adjacent intraepithelial disease [4].

Following the use of sentinel lymph node biopsy in assessing prognosis of cutaneous melanomas, its use has also been considered for patients with conjunctival melanoma [55]. It is not yet known whether sentinel node biopsy influences the outcome, so that this procedure is mostly viewed as a prognostic one. A population-based analysis suggested that lymph node metastasis is not frequent enough to justify a sentinel node biopsy if the primary tumor is limbal and < 2 mm in thickness [56].

Table 12.1 TNM staging

Category	Clinical classification	Pathologic classification
TX	Primary tumor cannot be assessed	Primary tumor cannot be assessed
T0	No evidence of primary tumor	No evidence of primary tumor
Tis	Melanoma in situ	Melanoma confined to conjunctival epithelium
T1: bulbar conjunctiva		
T1a	<1 quadrant in size	Invasion of substantia propria, ≤2 mm thickness
T1b	≥1 to <2 quadrants in size	Invasion of substantia propria, >2 mm thickness
T1c	≥2 to <3 quadrants in size	–
T1d	≥3 quadrants in size	–
T2: Non-bulbar conjunctiva (palpebral, forniceal, tarsal) and caruncular		
T2a	Non-caruncular and ≤ 1 quadrant of non-bulbar conjunctiva	Invasion of substantia propria, ≤2 mm thickness
T2b	Non-caruncular and > 1 quadrant of non-bulbar conjunctiva	Invasion of substantia propria, >2 mm thickness
T2c	Caruncular and ≤ 1 quadrant of non-bulbar conjunctiva	–
T2d	Caruncular and > 1 quadrant of non-bulbar conjunctiva	–
T3: Local invasion (globe, orbit, eyelid, nasolacrimal system, or sinuses)		
T3a	Globe involved	Globe involved
T3b	Eyelid involved	Eyelid involved
T3c	Orbit involved	Orbit involved
T3d	Nasolacrimal duct, lacrimal sac, and/or paranasal sinus	Nasolacrimal duct, lacrimal sac, and/or paranasal sinus
T4: Central nervous system invasion (any size)		
T4	Central nervous system involved	Central nervous system involved

Regional Lymph Node
NX: Regional lymph nodes cannot be assessed
N0: No regional lymph node metastasis
N1: Regional lymph node metastasis
Metastasis
M0: No distant metastasis
M1: Distant metastasis
Data from Jain et al. (2019) [54]

Management

Advances in cryotherapy, radiotherapy, and chemothcrapy for CoM have decreased the need for exenteration [57]. Primary tumors are excised following a "no touch" surgical approach to remove the entire tumor and minimize the risk of recurrence and metastasis [24, 57]. It is hypothesized that inadequate surgical methods lead to recurrence and metastasis likely through iatrogenic seeding of tumor; therefore fresh sterile instruments are suggested to be used at each step [19, 24]. Margins of 2 mm are required, though some surgeons attempt to include 5–7 mm margins when possible [24].

The surgical approach has been described previously [57]. First, the conjunctival incision lines are marked on the conjunctiva with bipolar diathermy, which also prevents hemorrhage. If the tumor extends to the limbus, then the affected corneal epithelium is debrided using alcohol and a Bard–Parker knife. Using blunt-tipped spring scissors, the tumor is excised, ensuring meticulous hemostasis. Any adhesion to the sclera is treated with bipolar diathermy, leaving the sclera surface intact. The corneal part of the tumor is dissected with a Bard–Parker knife to include the debrided, affected corneal epithelium. Just before the excision is completed, the specimen is placed on a paper mount, stabilized by a narrow bridge of tissues, which also prevents scrolling. Using fresh instruments, the conjunctiva is undermined and closed with interrupted, absorbable sutures.

To reduce the risk of recurrence, it is recommended that conjunctival margins are treated with double freeze-thaw cryotherapy with the conjunctiva raised to avoid damage to the sclera [19].

Another possibility is adjunctive brachytherapy applied using a 15-mm ruthenium plaque and administering a dose of 100 Gy to a depth of 1 mm after the conjunctiva has healed. If there is diffuse, lateral, intra-epithelial spread or underlying C-MIN, then adjunctive topical chemotherapy with mitomycin C is administered. Lamellar sclera excision is not performed, which causes an unsightly scar and may increase the chances of melanoma recurrence in this area, with possible intraocular infiltration. An amniotic membrane graft is only rarely necessary. The brachytherapy is administered even if histology suggests complete surgical clearance, as conventional sectioning may have missed the deepest part of the tumor. If the tumor involves the fornix or caruncular area, then proton-beam radiotherapy is administered [57].

In extensive disease, when the eye cannot be salvaged, orbital exenteration with or without adjuvant radiotherapy is required [26]. Unfortunately, some studies have suggested that this is only palliative, not having any effect on survival [58].

Up to 50% of the patients with systemic metastases show regional lymph node involvement before systemic involvement [56]. However, the use of sentinel lymph node biopsy (SLNB) for staging the disease and identifying patients with micro nodal metastasis is controversial [59–61]. Twenty-six percent of the patients with regional metastases never develop systemic disease [62]. SLNB has shown benefit in the ocular adnexal tumors of 2 mm thickness or more but may be useful in less thick tumors if associated with ulceration [61]. Furthermore, there is no consensus about when this should be performed, and in whom, and the technique requires special expertise [63].

Screening patients with CoM who are at elevated risk of metastasis involves a full medical examination including ophthalmological exam and palpation of head and neck lymph nodes, chest radiography, liver ultrasound scans and liver function tests, performed every 6 months for 10 years and is undertaken routinely in some centers [19]. Although the role of positron emission tomography (PET) is still uncertain [60], whole-body PET/CT has been reported to be superior to routine radiographic imaging modalities in detecting systemic metastasis, specifically bone involvement, but its use is limited by its prohibitive cost, false negative results, and nonspecificity [64].

Evidence is emerging that metastatic CoM may respond to treatments for metastatic cutaneous melanoma, such as targeted therapy and immunotherapy [65]. In a study of 27 primary conjunctival melanoma patients, 5 (19%) had PD-L1 expression and were associated with more distant metastases [66]. One report of five patients treated with nivolumab or pembrolizumab showed that four had no evidence of disease at 1 to 36 months after completion of treatment and one patient had stable disease [66]. A couple of other studies report patients with resolution after anti-PD-1 therapy [2–4, 67–69]. Adverse effects from immunotherapy are generally autoimmune and inflammatory, affecting the skin, liver, GI tract, respiratory tract, nervous system, and endocrine systems. It is also noted that ocular complications such as uveitis can arise, possibly due to a role of PD-L1 has in maintaining the eye's immune privilege [66].

Prognosis

Institution- and population-based retrospective studies [21, 26, 70–72] have consistently shown that the location and size of the primary conjunctival melanoma are strong and independent predictors of prognosis. Patients with primary tumors located at the limbus, their most common site, or displaced to the cornea [8] carry a better prognosis than tumors located in the forniceal conjunctiva, caruncle, plica semilunaris, or eyelid margins [26, 57].

Local tumor recurrence is reported to occur in more than 50% of these cases [21, 71, 73]. Risk factors for recurrence are reported to be multifocal disease, non-limbal position of the tumor, involvement of the surgical margin, and surgical excision without adjunctive treatment [26, 74]. Studies have shown lower rates of recurrence when patients are routinely administered adjunctive radiotherapy irrespective of histological clearance [57]. The mean time to recurrence is estimated to be 2.5 years.

Metastatic disease develops in 20–30% of patients [4, 26, 71]. Clinical risk factors include disease recurrence, involvement of non-bulbar conjunctiva, medial bulbar conjunctiva, caruncle and plica semilunaris, and tumor thickness of more than 2 mm [21, 26, 56, 58, 68, 75]. Poor prognostic histopathologic features comprise high mitotic count, presence of epithelioid cells, diffuse intraepithelial disease, extravascular matrix pattern, and surface ulceration [10, 26, 76]. CoM arising de novo is associated with a higher risk of metastases and death, compared to tumors arising from a nevus or PAM [19].

There is compelling circumstantial evidence correlating local tumor recurrence with metastasis [4, 26, 71]. In 45–60% of cases, the first site for metastasis is the regional lymph nodes, specifically the periauricular, submandibular, or cervical lymph nodes, developing after a median of 2.3 years [77]. Systemic disease most commonly involves lungs, brain, liver, skin, bones, and gastrointestinal tract and is typically detected at a median of 3.4 years [74]. The estimated 5-year mortality of

CoM is 12–19%, whereas the 10-year mortality rate is around 30% [1, 21, 23, 26, 75].

The rarity of CoM has traditionally complicated understanding of the disease. However, recent advances in stratifying risk and in treatment technique have improved outcomes for patients. Furthermore, the similarities between CoM and cutaneous melanoma may allow its inclusion into more clinical trials.

References

1. Seregard S. Conjunctival melanoma. Surv Ophthalmol. 1998;42(4):321–50.
2. Brownstein S. Malignant melanoma of the conjunctiva. Cancer Control. 2004;11(5):310–6.
3. Grossniklaus HE, Green WR, Luckenbach M, Chan CC. Conjunctival lesions in adults: a clinical and histopathologic review. Cornea. 1987;6(2):78.
4. Damato B, Coupland SE. Conjunctival melanoma and melanosis: a reappraisal of terminology, classification and staging. Clin Experiment Ophthalmol. 2008;36(8):786–95.
5. Shields JA, Shields CL, Mashayekhi A, Marr BP, Benavides R, Thangappan A, et al. Primary acquired melanosis of the conjunctiva: experience with 311 eyes. Trans Am Ophthalmol Soc. 2007;105:61–72.
6. Jakobiec FA, Folberg R, Iwamoto T. Clinicopathologic characteristics of premalignant and malignant melanocytic lesions of the conjunctiva. Ophthalmology. 1989;96(2):147–66.
7. Paridaens AD, McCartney AC, Hungerford JL. Multifocal amelanotic conjunctival melanoma and acquired melanosis sine pigmento. Br J Ophthalmol. 1992;76(3):163–5.
8. Tuomaala S, Aine E, Saari KM, Kivelä T. Corneally displaced malignant conjunctival melanomas. Ophthalmology. 2002;109(5):914–9.
9. Shields JA, Shields CL, Mashayekhi A, Marr BP, Benavides R, Thangappan A, et al. Primary acquired melanosis of the conjunctiva: risks for progression to melanoma in 311 eyes: the 2006 Lorenz E. Zimmerman Lecture. Ophthalmology. 2008;115(3):511–9.e2
10. Damato B, Coupland SE. Management of conjunctival melanoma. Expert Rev Anticancer Ther. 2009;9(9):1227–39.
11. Jakobiec FA, Rini FJ, Fraunfelder FT, Brownstein S. Cryotherapy for conjunctival primary acquired melanosis and malignant melanoma: experience with 62 cases. Ophthalmology. 1988;95(8):1058–70.
12. Paridaens D, Beekhuis H, van den Bosch W, Remeyer L, Melles G. Amniotic membrane transplantation in the management of conjunctival malignant melanoma and primary acquired melanosis with atypia. Br J Ophthalmol. 2001;85(6):658–61.
13. Kurli M, Finger PT. Topical mitomycin chemotherapy for conjunctival malignant melanoma and primary acquired melanosis with atypia: 12 years' experience. Graefe's Arch Clin Exp Ophthalmol. 2005;243(11):1108–14.
14. Pe'er J, Frucht-Pery J. The treatment of primary acquired melanosis (PAM) with atypia by topical Mitomycin C. Am J Ophthalmol. 2005;139(2):229–34.
15. Finger PT, Sedeek RW, Chin KJ. Topical interferon alfa in the treatment of conjunctival melanoma and primary acquired melanosis complex. Am J Ophthalmol. 2008;145(1):124–9.e1
16. Frucht-Pery J, Pe'er J. Use of Mitomycin C in the treatment of conjunctival primary acquired melanosis with atypia. Arch Ophthalmol. 1996;114(10):1261–4.
17. Folberg R, McLean IW, Zimmerman LE. Malignant melanoma of the conjunctiva. Hum Pathol. 1985;16(2):136–43.
18. Isager P, Østerlind A, Engholm G, Heegaard S, Lindegaard J, Overgaard J, et al. Uveal and conjunctival malignant melanoma in Denmark, 1943–97: incidence and validation study. Ophthalmic Epidemiol. 2005;12(4):223–32.

19. Kaštelan S, Gverović Antunica A, Beketić Orešković L, Salopek Rabatić J, Kasun B, Bakija I. Conjunctival melanoma—epidemiological trends and features. Pathol Oncol Res. 2018;24(4):787–96.
20. Folberg R, McLean IW, Zimmerman LE. Primary acquired melanosis of the conjunctiva. Hum Pathol. 1985;16(2):129–35.
21. Missotten GS, Keijser S, Keizer RJWD, Wolff-Rouendaal DD. Conjunctival melanoma in The Netherlands: a Nationwide study. Invest Ophthalmol Vis Sci. 2005;46(1):75–82.
22. Shields CL, Fasiudden A, Mashayekhi A, Shields JA. Conjunctival nevi: clinical features and natural course in 410 consecutive patients. Arch Ophthalmol. 2004;122(2):167–75.
23. Kurli M, Finger PT. Melanocytic conjunctival tumors. Ophthalmol Clin. 2005;18(1):15–24.
24. Vora GK, Demirci H, Marr B, Mruthyunjaya P. Advances in the management of conjunctival melanoma. Surv Ophthalmol. 2017;62(1):26–42.
25. McDonnell JM, Carpenter JD, Jacobs P, Wan WL, Gilmore JE. Conjunctival melanocytic lesions in children. Ophthalmology. 1989;96(7):986–93.
26. Shields CL, Shields JA, Gündüz K, Cater J, Mercado GV, Gross N, et al. Conjunctival melanoma: risk factors for recurrence, exenteration, metastasis, and death in 150 consecutive patients. Arch Ophthalmol. 2000;118(11):1497–507.
27. Mohamed MD, Gupta M, Parsons A, Rennie IG. Ultrasound biomicroscopy in the management of melanocytoma of the ciliary body with extrascleral extension. Br J Ophthalmol. 2005;89(1):14–6.
28. Kiratli H, Shields CL, Shields JA, DePotter P. Metastatic tumours to the conjunctiva: report of 10 cases. Br J Ophthalmol. 1996;80(1):5–8.
29. Spendlove HE, Damato BE, Humphreys J, Barker KT, Hiscott PS, Houlston RS. BRAF mutations are detectable in conjunctival but not uveal melanomas. Melanoma Res. 2004;14(6):449.
30. Gear H, Williams H, Kemp EG, Roberts F. BRAF mutations in conjunctival melanoma. Invest Ophthalmol Vis Sci. 2004;45(8):2484–8.
31. Davies H, Bignell GR, Cox C, Stephens P, Edkins S, Clegg S, et al. Mutations of the BRAF gene in human cancer. Nature. 2002;417(6892):949–54.
32. Lake SL, Jmor F, Dopierala J, Taktak AFG, Coupland SE, Damato BE. Multiplex ligation-dependent probe amplification of conjunctival melanoma reveals common BRAF V600E gene mutation and gene copy number changes. Invest Ophthalmol Vis Sci. 2011;52(8):5598–604.
33. Chapman PB, Hauschild A, Robert C, Haanen JB, Ascierto P, Larkin J, et al. Improved survival with vemurafenib in melanoma with BRAF V600E mutation. N Engl J Med. 2011;364(26):2507–16.
34. Kiyohara T, Tanimura H, Miyamoto M, Shijimaya T, Nagano N, Nakamaru S, et al. Two cases of BRAF-mutated, bulbar conjunctival melanoma, and review of the published literature. Clin Exp Dermatol. 2020;45(2):207–11.
35. Mor JM, Heindl LM. Systemic BRAF/MEK inhibitors as a potential treatment option in metastatic conjunctival melanoma. Ocul Oncol Pathol. 2017;3(2):133–41.
36. Kim JM, Weiss S, Sinard JH, Pointdujour-Lim R. Dabrafenib and trametinib for BRAF-mutated conjunctival melanoma. Ocul Oncol Pathol. 2020;6(1):35–8.
37. Lami H, Epstein RJ, Cherepanoff S, Conway RM. Effective conservative management of locally advanced conjunctival melanoma using initial systemic therapy. Clin Experiment Ophthalmol. 2020;48(3):402–4.
38. de Keizer PLJ, Packer LM, Szypowska AA, Riedl-Polderman PE, van den Broek NJF, de Bruin A, et al. Activation of FOXO transcription factors by oncogenic BRAF promotes p21cip1-dependent senescence. Cancer Res. 2010;70(21):8526–36.
39. Shamloo U. p21 in cancer research. Cancers. 2019;11(8):1178.
40. Packer LM, Pavey SJ, Boyle GM, Stark MS, Ayub AL, Rizos H, et al. Gene expression profiling in melanoma identifies novel downstream effectors of p14ARF. Int J Cancer. 2007;121(4):784–90.
41. Jiang H, Lin J, Su Z, Herlyn M, Kerbel R, Weissman B, et al. The melanoma differentiation-associated gene mda-6, which encodes the cyclin-dependent kinase inhibitor p21, is

differentially expressed during growth, differentiation and progression in human melanoma cells. Oncogene. 1995;10:1855–64.
42. Riminucci M, Corsi A, Peris K, Fisher LW, Chimenti S, Bianco P. Coexpression of bone sialoprotein (BSP) and the pivotal transcriptional regulator of osteogenesis, Cbfa1/Runx2, in malignant melanoma. Calcif Tissue Int. 2003;73(3):281–9.
43. Baniwal SK, Khalid O, Gabet Y, Shah RR, Purcell DJ, Mav D, et al. Runx2 transcriptome of prostate cancer cells: insights into invasiveness and bone metastasis. Mol Cancer. 2010;9:258.
44. Leong DT, Lim J, Goh X, Pratap J, Pereira BP, Kwok HS, et al. Cancer-related ectopic expression of the bone-related transcription factor RUNX2 in non-osseous metastatic tumor cells is linked to cell proliferation and motility. Breast Cancer Res. 2010;12(5):R89.
45. Bornfeld N, Prescher G, Becher R, Hirche H, Jöckel K-H, Horsthemke B. Prognostic implications of monosomy 3 in uveal melanoma. Lancet. 1996;347(9010):1222–5.
46. Mensink HW, Kiliç E, Vaarwater J, Douben H, Paridaens D, de Klein A. Molecular cytogenetic analysis of archival uveal melanoma with known clinical outcome. Cancer Genet Cytogenet. 2008;181(2):108–11.
47. Kilic E, Naus NC, van Gils W, Klaver CC, van Til ME, Verbiest MM, et al. Concurrent loss of chromosome arm 1p and chromosome 3 predicts a decreased disease-free survival in uveal melanoma patients. Invest Ophthalmol Vis Sci. 2005;46(7):2253–7.
48. McNamara M, Felix C, Val Davison E, Fenton M, Kennedy SM. Assessment of chromosome 3 copy number in ocular melanoma using fluorescence in situ hybridization. Cancer Genet Cytogenet. 1997;98(1):4–8.
49. Sobin LH, Fleming ID. TNM classification of malignant tumors, fifth edition (1997). Cancer. 1997;80(9):1803–4.
50. Sobin LH, Wittekind C. TNM Classification of Malignant Tumours, 6th edition | UICC [Internet]. [cited 2019 Sep 14]. Available from: https://www.uicc.org/resources/tnm-classification-malignant-tumours-6th-edition
51. Edge SB. American joint committee on cancer, editors. AJCC cancer staging manual. 7th ed. New York: Springer; 2010. 648.
52. Yousef YA, Finger PT. Predictive value of the seventh edition American Joint Committee on Cancer Staging System for Conjunctival Melanoma. Arch Ophthalmol. 2012;130(5):599–606.
53. Shields C, Kaliki S, Al-Dahmash S, Lally S, Shields J. American joint committee on cancer (AJCC) clinical classification predicts conjunctival melanoma outcomes. Ophthalmic Plast Reconstr Surg. 2012;28(5):313–23.
54. Jain P, Finger PT, Damato B, Coupland SE, Heimann H, Kenawy N, et al. Multicenter, international assessment of the eighth edition of the American Joint Committee on Cancer Staging Manual for Conjunctival Melanoma. JAMA Ophthalmol. 2019;137(8):905–11.
55. Esmaeli B, Eicher S, Popp J, Delpassand E, Prieto VG, Gershenwald JE. Sentinel lymph node biopsy for conjunctival melanoma. Ophthalmic Plast Reconstr Surg. 2001;17(6):436.
56. Tuomaala S, Kivelä T. Metastatic pattern and survival in disseminated conjunctival melanoma: implications for sentinel lymph node biopsy. Ophthalmology. 2004;111(4):816–21.
57. Damato B, Coupland SE. An audit of conjunctival melanoma treatment in Liverpool. Eye. 2009;23(4):801–9.
58. Paridaens AD, McCartney AC, Minassian DC, Hungerford JL. Orbital exenteration in 95 cases of primary conjunctival malignant melanoma. Br J Ophthalmol. 1994;78(7):520–8.
59. Tuomaala S, Kivelä T. Sentinel lymph node biopsy guidelines for conjunctival melanoma. Melanoma Research [Internet]. 2008;18:3. Jun [cited 2019 Sep 12]. Available from: https://journals.lww.com/melanomaresearch/Citation/2008/06000/Sentinel_lymph_node_biopsy_guidelines_for.12.aspx
60. Esmaeli B. Regional lymph node assessment for conjunctival melanoma: sentinel lymph node biopsy and positron emission tomography. Br J Ophthalmol. 2008;92(4):443–5.
61. Savar A, Ross MI, Prieto VG, Ivan D, Kim S, Esmaeli B. Sentinel lymph node biopsy for ocular adnexal melanoma: experience in 30 patients. Ophthalmology. 2009;116(11):2217–23.

62. Esmaeli B, Wang X, Youssef A, Gershenwald JE. Patterns of regional and distant metastasis in patients with conjunctival melanoma: experience at a cancer center over four decades. Ophthalmology. 2001;108(11):2101–5.
63. Morton DL, Thompson JF, Cochran AJ, Mozzillo N, Elashoff R, Essner R, et al. Sentinel-node biopsy or nodal observation in melanoma. N Engl J Med. 2006;355(13):1307–17.
64. Patel P, Finger PT. Whole-body 18F FDG positron emission tomography/computed tomography evaluation of patients with uveal metastasis. Am J Ophthalmol. 2012;153(4):661–8.
65. Grimes JM, Shah NV, Samie FH, Carvajal RD, Marr BP. Conjunctival melanoma: current treatments and future options. Am J Clin Dermatol. 2020;21(3):371–81.
66. Lu JE, Chang JR, Berry JL, In GK, Zhang-Nunes S. Clinical update on checkpoint inhibitor therapy for conjunctival and eyelid melanoma. Int Ophthalmol Clin. 2020;60(2):77–89.
67. Chaves LJ, Huth B, Augsburger JJ, Correa ZM. Eye-sparing treatment for diffuse invasive conjunctival melanoma. Ocul Oncol Pathol. 2018;4(4):261–6.
68. Kini A, Fu R, Compton C, Miller DM, Ramasubramanian A. Pembrolizumab for recurrent conjunctival melanoma. JAMA Ophthalmol. 2017;135(8):891–2.
69. Pinto Torres S, André T, Gouveia E, Costa L, Passos MJ. Systemic treatment of metastatic conjunctival melanoma. Case Rep Oncol Med. 2017;2017:4623964.
70. Tuomaala S, Eskelin S, Tarkkanen A, Kivelä T. Population-based assessment of clinical characteristics predicting outcome of conjunctival melanoma in whites. Invest Ophthalmol Vis Sci. 2002;43(11):3399–408.
71. Anastassiou G, Heiligenhaus A, Bechrakis N, Bader E, Bornfeld N, Steuhl K-P. Prognostic value of clinical and histopathological parameters in conjunctival melanomas: a retrospective study. Br J Ophthalmol. 2002;86(2):163–7.
72. Norregaard JC, Gerner N, Jensen OA, Prause JU. Malignant melanoma of the conjunctiva: occurrence and survival following surgery and radiotherapy in a Danish population. Graefes Arch Clin Exp Ophthalmol. 1996;234(9):569–72.
73. Shields JA, Shields CL, Gündüz K, Cater J. Clinical features predictive of orbital exenteration for conjunctival melanoma. Ophthalmic Plast Reconstr Surg. 2000;16(3):173.
74. De Potter P, Shields CL, Shields JA, Menduke H. Clinical predictive factors for development of recurrence and metastasis in conjunctival melanoma: a review of 68 cases. Br J Ophthalmol. 1993;77(10):624–30.
75. Paridaens AD, Minassian DC, McCartney AC, Hungerford JL. Prognostic factors in primary malignant melanoma of the conjunctiva: a clinicopathological study of 256 cases. Br J Ophthalmol. 1994;78(4):252–9.
76. Tuomaala S, Toivonen P, Al-Jamal R, Kivelä T. Prognostic significance of histopathology of primary conjunctival melanoma in Caucasians. Curr Eye Res. 2007;32(11):939–52.
77. Folberg R, McLean IW. Primary acquired melanosis and melanoma of the conjunctiva: terminology, classification, and biologic behavior. Human Pathol. 1986;17(7):652–4.

Minority Melanoma Paradox

13

While melanoma is uncommon in patients of African, Hispanic, and Asian descent, it is frequently fatal for these populations [1]. The incidence of melanoma is 45.8 diagnoses per 100,000 in non-Hispanic Whites (NHW); 6.8 for Hispanics; 5.72 for the group consisting of Asians, Native Americans, and Pacific Islanders; and 1.35 for Blacks [2]. Despite this, melanomas among minority populations are more likely to be diagnosed at an advanced stage, metastasize, and have poorer outcomes than among NHW (Fig. 13.1).

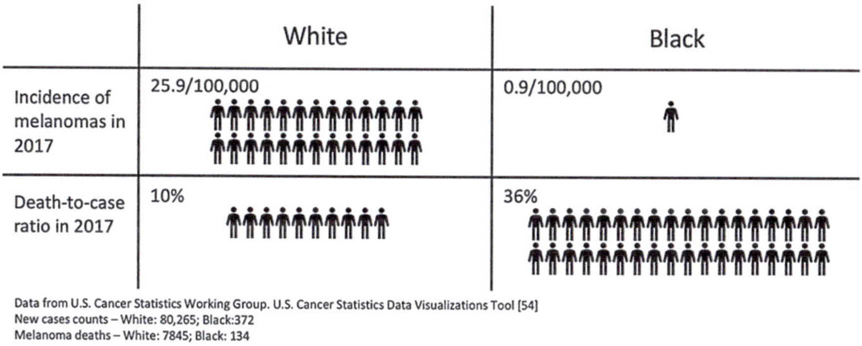
White
Black
Incidence of melanomas in 2017
25.9/100,000
0.9/100,000
Death-to-case ratio in 2017
10%
36%
Data from U.S. Cancer Statistics Working Group. U.S. Cancer Statistics Data Visualizations Tool [54]
New cases counts – White: 80,265; Black:372
Melanoma deaths – White: 7845; Black: 134

Fig. 13.1 Incidences and rates of melanoma death in White and Black populations in the United States [54]

S. Ortiz-Urda et al., *Melanoma*, https://doi.org/10.1007/978-3-031-59128-0_13

Melanoma Development in Non-White Populations

Although many studies demonstrate the trend of minority populations having a lower incidence of melanoma and having more advanced disease at diagnosis, the etiology remains poorly understood [3]. The lower incidence of melanoma in Hispanics and Black individuals has been partially attributed to the protective advantage of a higher Fitzpatrick skin type on average [4]. Specifically, darker skin has increased melanin density and melanosomal distribution [4]. The number of melanocytes remains the same; however, the product of melanocytes—melanin—tends to be larger and more widely distributed. With increased melanin content, the larger melanosomes of darker skin absorb and scatter more energy than the smaller melanosomes of lighter skin. The epidermis of Black individuals has a natural sun protection factor of 13.4, effectively filtering twice as much UVB radiation as the epidermis of Caucasians [5]. There is a significant correlation between the absolute amount and distribution of melanin and the amount of photoprotection from UV-induced DNA damage [6].

Although melanin plays a significant role in protection, the risk for melanoma is not eliminated. Melanoma is associated with increased UV radiation exposure in all races including African Americans and Hispanics [7]. As with NHW, the incidence of melanoma has been increasing for all other ethnic groups and has been attributed to continued ozone depletion, upward social mobility and subsequent increase in outdoor leisurely sun exposure and travel to lower latitudes, and increased intermittent sun exposure [5, 8–11]. Although many ethnic minorities sustain chronic UV exposure from jobs in the labor force such as agriculture and construction, individuals exposed to intermittent UV exposure from recreational activity have been described to be at higher risk than outdoor workers [12].

There are likely many risk factors other than UV radiation that affect melanoma development in minority groups, as most cases develop in areas of the body that are not regularly sun-exposed [13–15]. Studying genetic alterations of melanoma in different anatomical locations, several researchers have explored the theory that melanoma is a heterogenous disease with varying etiologies [16, 17]. Incidence patterns seem to be specific by anatomical site [18]. Whitman et al. in 2003 developed the "divergent pathway" model to explain the variation observed [17]. They hypothesized that individuals with high melanocyte proliferation are more likely to develop melanoma with less or intermittent UV radiation exposure on sites like the trunk [17]. Other individuals with low melanocyte proliferation seem to require chronic UV exposure for melanoma to develop [17].

Environmental exposure to carcinogens has been proposed as a risk factor. Although ethnic minorities have in large part been omitted from occupational investigations [19], one study reported increased mortality from melanoma among African American women employed in the machinery and transportation equipment-manufacturing sector [20]. Of note, malignant melanoma has been associated with exposure to polychlorinated biphenyls (PCBs) in both the machinery and transportation equipment manufacturing industries [21, 22].

Significant gaps in knowledge remain of how melanin density, melanin distribution, and DNA damage and repair mechanisms among individuals with different ethnic origins affect melanoma risk. Analysis of melanoma incidence data in Hispanics and African Americans is limited by the low incidence in these populations and the traditional lack of cancer data for Hispanic patients who were not identified by ethnic category in state cancer registries [23, 24]. Although identification of these cases has improved, the number of cases remains underestimated [25, 26].

Melanoma is more often diagnosed at a later stage in African American patients than for NHW patients. Moreover, 75.9% of melanoma in NHW patients were diagnosed at Stage I, while in African American patients, this was only 52.6% [2]. Conversely, 32–52% of melanomas in African Americans were diagnosed at Stage III/IV, compared to just 12–16% of NHW patients [27, 28]. A study of NCDB data analyzing the odds for a cohort of 157,308 melanoma patients diagnosed between 2004 and 2013 found that African American patients were 4.81 times more likely than NHW patients to be diagnosed at Stage IV [29]. Similarly, Hispanic melanoma patients are more likely to present with Stage III disease and 3.64 (CI: 2.65–5.0) times more likely to have distant metastases than non-Hispanic Whites [4, 27]. Asian and Pacific Islander patients may present with advanced disease at an even higher rate, with 55% having regional or remote involvement [30].

The overall 5-year melanoma survival rate for African Americans hovers around 77% versus 91% for Caucasians [31]. One analysis of data from the National Cancer Institute's Surveillance, Epidemiology, and End Result (SEER) program found that non-Hispanic Black patients have a cause-specific mortality hazard ratio of 2.5 compared to the reference group of non-Hispanic Whites after adjusting for site of diagnosis, gender, age, and decade of diagnosis [32]. However, after substituting stage of diagnosis for site in the adjustments, the cause-specific mortality hazard ratio dropped to 0.7, demonstrating the importance of the melanoma stage [32]. Another study of SEER data from 1992 to 2009 shows that the melanoma mortality by stage in African Americans compared to Whites is only significantly higher in Stage I and Stage III, non-significantly higher in Stage II melanoma, and there was no difference in stage IV melanoma [2]. The largest differences probably reflect the timeframe when valuable interventions are possible. A Fine and Gray competing risks regression model of SEER data found that Asian and Pacific Islander melanoma patients have a melanoma-specific mortality hazard ratio of 1.27 (95% CI: 1.12–1.43) and overall mortality hazard ratio of 1.17 (95% CI: 1.07–1.28) compared to White patients with melanoma [33].

Clinical Presentation

While 90% of Caucasian melanoma patients developed a tumor on skin that is regularly sun-exposed, only 33% of African American patients developed melanoma in these areas [15]. The most common sun-protected sites where melanoma develops include the foot, palmar and plantar surfaces, toenails, mucous membranes of the mouth, nasal passages, or genitals [34]. Melanomas in African Americans, Asians, Filipinos, Indonesians, and native Hawaiians most often occur on non-exposed skin with less pigment, with up to 60–75% of tumors arising on the palms, soles, mucous membranes, and nail regions [35]. The lower extremity was the most common anatomical location reported for minorities [36]: the foot among Black Americans [37] and the leg among Hispanic Americans [38]. Other rare presentations have also been reported in higher rates in African American patients including those originating on the buttocks, nasal cavity, and congenital nevi [27].

When melanoma occurs in African Americans, a different histological subtype predominates. While superficial spreading melanoma is the most common histological subtype reported among Hispanics and Whites [37], acral lentiginous melanoma is the most common melanoma growth pattern (60%) reported among African Americans and Asians [34, 39]. Acral lentiginous melanoma in African American patients usually presents at an advanced clinical and histopathologic stage with an expected poor prognosis. It appears as an unevenly and dark brown pigmented patch on sun-protected areas of the skin [27]. The course of the disease and the outcome of treatment of these patients are poorly documented [40]. Primary melanoma tumors among African Americans are commonly misdiagnosed and treated as a plantar wart, tinea nigra, or talon noir [41]. Comparing survival rates between African Americans and NHW with melanoma of the same stage and medical treatment, survival rates were still lower for African Americans. One retrospective review in California also found a higher proportion of acral lentiginous melanomas among Hispanic males (5.1%) vs. White males (0.6%) [42]. A greater proportion of melanomas in minority populations were also found to be mucosal rather than cutaneous [30]. Mucosal melanomas show a preferential anatomical distribution by racial groups with anorectal melanomas most common in Asian patients and genitourinary melanomas in NHW and Black patients [30]. The greater proportion of acral and mucosal melanoma, which exhibit more tumor growth because of a more virulent and aggressive nature, in minority populations likely contributes to the increased mortality rate.

In Asians, lesions were found to appear initially as a pigmented macule that progress to a rapidly expanding plaque with irregular, notched borders and may be ulcerated [39]. Subungual melanomas in Asians often begin as a brown or black discoloration of the nail and frequently becomes a well-demarcated, pigmented longitudinal streak before spreading and damaging the nail plate [39].

Breslow thickness correlates with mortality rates, and minorities are more likely to present with thicker melanoma tumors at diagnosis [27, 39]. The average Breslow thickness found in Asians was 4.9 mm compared to 2.0 mm for Whites [39, 43]. An analysis of melanoma data from the California Cancer reported that the incidence of invasive melanoma increased markedly among Hispanics in California compared to non-Hispanics and that thicker melanomas accounted for most of the increase [42, 44]. An analysis from the New Mexico Melanoma Registry and New Mexico Tumor Registry found that 36% of Hispanics melanoma patients had tumors 2 mm or thicker in depth, whereas only 16% of NHW melanoma patients had such advanced lesions [23] (Figs. 13.2 and 13.3).

Prevention

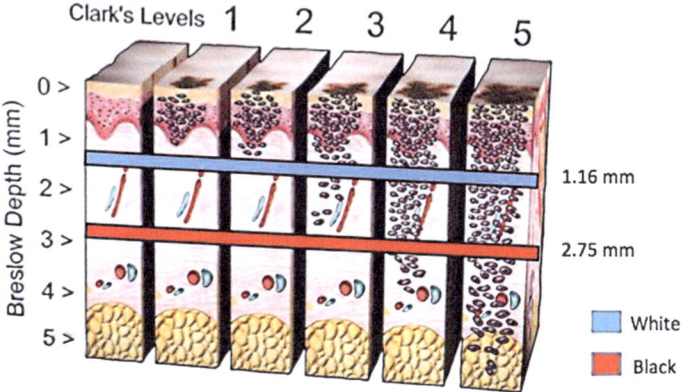

Fig. 13.2 Mean Breslow depth on presentation is 1.16 mm for White patients and 2.75 mm for Black patients [55]

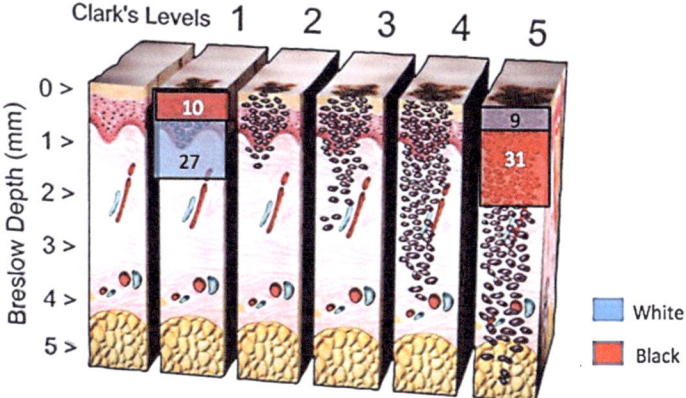

Fig. 13.3 Clark level 1: 10% of lesions in Black patients; 27% of lesions in White patients. Clark level 5: 31% of lesions in Black patients; 9% of lesions in White patients [28]

There remain just a limited number of published reports of characteristics of melanoma in minority populations in the United States [4, 45–47]. As the understanding of the characteristics of melanoma in these groups improves, physicians can be keener on making the appropriate interventions.

Prevention

While prevention measures with earlier detection may account for improved survival rates in White populations, similar advances have not been shown for other races [3]. The more advanced stage of melanoma at presentation in Hispanic and Black patients highlights the disparity in secondary prevention of melanoma in minority populations. According to the National Health Interview Surveys among US adults, both Hispanic and Black people are screened for skin cancer less frequently than are NHW [48]. Secondary prevention efforts such as skin cancer screenings are suboptimal in Hispanic and Black individuals [28]. The increasing incidence among these patients emphasizes the need for improved sun protection and risk education among these populations [35].

It is important for patients of minority backgrounds and their physicians to be cognizant that melanoma can and does occur in these groups. Greater efforts need to be made to inform these individuals about this potentially life-threatening but avoidable condition. In addition to sun protection, patients should be instructed in performing skin self-examinations with special emphasis on the feet, hands, nails, the area between the fingers and toes, and other non-sun-exposed areas and to immediately visit their dermatologist if they notice anything suspicious. Specifically, suspicious features commonly found are brown or black bands under the nails of the thumbs or big toes that extend into the nail folds or the skin that supports the nail.

Socioeconomic status, sociocultural values, and skin cancer awareness are likely factors that account for differences in the delivery and utilization of health-care resources among minority populations [1, 49, 50]. Poverty and lack of health insurance influence access and utilization of cancer screening services and treatment, thus contributing to current disparities in the cancer burden among minority groups [51, 52]. Compared to patients with private insurance, patients had significantly higher odds of Stage IV melanoma if they had Medicare (OR = 1.31, CI: 1.19–1.45), government insurance (OR = 2.19, CI: 1.61–2.98), Medicaid (OR = 6.97, CI: 5.98–8.13), or no insurance (OR = 5.10, CI: 4.41–5.91) [29]. Future considerations should be given to help meet the gap in access to care.

Among US racial and ethnic groups, African Americans carry the highest cancer burden. The disparities in the stage of diagnosis and survival rates of various cancers reflect an unequal access to health care [19]. Lastly, the delayed diagnosis of melanoma among Hispanic and Black patients could also reflect lower skin cancer awareness [1]. Darker-skinned individuals perceive themselves as having low or no risk for melanoma or were unaware of skin cancer and melanoma [53]. One study comparing skin cancer awareness among Hispanics to non-Hispanics Whites with similar access to health care found that Hispanics had a lower level of perceived risk and awareness of melanoma and other skin cancers [46]. Lower skin cancer awareness could influence an individual's decision to delay seeking timely medical care for suspicious skin lesions.

Conclusion

The delayed presentation of melanoma and the lower survival rates among minority groups highlight an increasingly significant public health concern. The lowest survival rate and highest proportion of advanced presentation of melanoma are seen among Black patients. Most of the public knowledge of melanoma risk regards White populations, particularly those with blue eyes and blond or red hair. Public education regarding melanoma risk in Black and Hispanic patients and the delivery of skin cancer screening and examinations represents the main potential areas of intervention to improve diagnosis in minorities. We hope that earlier diagnosis of melanoma at a more favorable stage will ultimately improve melanoma survival in minority populations.

References

1. Goldenberg A, Vujic I, Sanlorenzo M, Ortiz-Urda S. Melanoma risk perception and prevention behavior among African-Americans: the minority melanoma paradox. Clin Cosmet Investig Dermatol. 2015;8:423–9.
2. Dawes SM, Tsai S, Gittleman H, Barnholtz-Sloan JS, Bordeaux JS. Racial disparities in melanoma survival. J Am Acad Dermatol. 2016;75(5):983–91.
3. SEER Cancer Statistics Review 1975–2004—Previous Version—SEER Cancer Statistics [Internet]. SEER. [cited 2019 Sep 11]. Available from: https://seer.cancer.gov/archive/csr/1975_2004/index.html
4. Cress RD, Holly EA. Incidence of cutaneous melanoma among non-Hispanic whites, Hispanics, Asians, and Blacks: an analysis of California cancer registry data, 1988-93. Cancer Causes Control. 1997;8(2):246–52.
5. Halder RM, Ara CJ. Skin cancer and photoaging in ethnic skin. Dermatol Clin. 2003;21(4):725–32. x
6. Tadokoro T, Kobayashi N, Zmudzka BZ, Ito S, Wakamatsu K, Yamaguchi Y, et al. UV-induced DNA damage and melanin content in human skin differing in racial/ethnic origin. FASEB J. 2003;17(9):1177–9.
7. Hu S, Ma F, Collado-Mesa F, Kirsner RS. UV radiation, latitude, and melanoma in US Hispanics and Blacks. Arch Dermatol. 2004;140(7):819–24.
8. Harrison RA, Haque AU, Roseman JM, Soong SJ. Socioeconomic characteristics and melanoma incidence. Ann Epidemiol. 1998;8(5):327–33.
9. Gallagher RP, Elwood JM, Threlfall WJ, Spinelli JJ, Fincham S, Hill GB. Socioeconomic status, sunlight exposure, and risk of malignant melanoma: the Western Canada melanoma study. J Natl Cancer Inst. 1987;79(4):647–52.
10. Lee PY, Silverman MK, Rigel DS, Vossaert KA, Kopf AW, Bart RS, et al. Level of education and the risk of malignant melanoma. J Am Acad Dermatol. 1992;26(1):59–63.
11. Reynolds P, Elkin EP, Layefsky ME, Lee GM. Cancer in California school employees, 1988–1992. Am J Ind Med. 1999;36(2):271–8.
12. Elwood JM, Jopson J. Melanoma and sun exposure: an overview of published studies. Int J Cancer. 1997;73(2):198–203.
13. Elder DE. Skin cancer. Melanoma and other specific nonmelanoma skin cancers. Cancer. 1995;75(1 Suppl):245–56.
14. Armstrong BK, Kricker A. How much melanoma is caused by sun exposure? Melanoma Res. 1993;3(6):395.
15. Katz RD, Potter GK, Slutskiy PZ, Smith RRL, Ptau RG, Berlin SJ. A statistical survey of melanomas of the foot. J Am Acad Dermatol. 1993;28(6):1008–11.
16. Curtin JA, Fridlyand J, Kageshita T, Patel HN, Busam KJ, Kutzner H, et al. Distinct sets of genetic alterations in melanoma. N Engl J Med. 2005;353(20):2135–47.
17. Whiteman DC, Watt P, Purdie DM, Hughes MC, Hayward NK, Green AC. Melanocytic nevi, solar keratoses, and divergent pathways to cutaneous melanoma. J Natl Cancer Inst. 2003;95(11):806–12.
18. Lachiewicz AM, Berwick M, Wiggins CL, Thomas NE. Epidemiologic support for melanoma heterogeneity using the surveillance, epidemiology, and end results program. J Invest Dermatol. 2008;128(5):1340–2.

19. Ghafoor A, Jemal A, Cokkinides V, Cardinez C, Murray T, Samuels A, et al. Cancer statistics for African Americans. CA Cancer J Clin. 2002;52(6):326–41.
20. Loomis D, Schulz M. Mortality from six work-related cancers among African Americans and Latinos. Am J Ind Med. 2000;38(5):565–75.
21. Loomis D, Browning SR, Schenck AP, Gregory E, Savitz DA. Cancer mortality among electric utility workers exposed to polychlorinated biphenyls. Occup Environ Med. 1997;54(10):720–8.
22. Sinks T, Steele G, Smith AB, Watkins K, Shults RA. Mortality among workers exposed to polychlorinated biphenyls. Am J Epidemiol. 1992;136(4):389–98.
23. Black WC, Goldhahn RT, Wiggins C. Melanoma within a southwestern Hispanic population. Arch Dermatol. 1987;123(10):1331–4.
24. Poe GS, Powell-Griner E, McLaughlin JK, Placek PJ, Thompson GB, Robinson K. Comparability of the death certificate and the 1986 National Mortality Followback Survey. Vital Health Stat 2. 1993;118:1–53.
25. Howe HL, Wu X, Ries LAG, Cokkinides V, Ahmed F, Jemal A, et al. Annual report to the nation on the status of cancer, 1975-2003, featuring cancer among U.S. Hispanic/Latino populations. Cancer. 2006;107(8):1711–42.
26. O'Brien K, Cokkinides V, Jemal A, Cardinez CJ, Murray T, Samuels A, et al. Cancer statistics for hispanics, 2003. CA: CA Cancer J Clin. 2003;53(4):208–26.
27. Higgins S, Nazemi A, Feinstein S, Chow M, Wysong A. Clinical presentations of melanoma in African Americans, Hispanics, and Asians. Dermatologic Surg. 2019;45(6):791–801.
28. Hu S, Soza-Vento RM, Parker DF, Kirsner RS. Comparison of stage at diagnosis of melanoma among Hispanic, Black, and white patients in Miami-Dade County, Florida. Arch Dermatol. 2006;142(6):704–8.
29. Dick M, Aurit S, Silberstein P. The odds of stage IV melanoma diagnoses based on socioeconomic factors. J Cutan Med Surg. 2019;23(4):421–7.
30. Altieri L, Wong MK, Peng DH, Cockburn M. Mucosal melanomas in the racially diverse population of California. J Am Acad Dermatol. 2017;76(2):250–7.
31. Jemal A, Siegel R, Xu J, Ward E. Cancer statistics, 2010. CA Cancer J Clin. 2010;60(5): 277–300.
32. Ward-Peterson M, Acuña JM, Alkhalifah MK, Nasiri AM, Al-Akeel ES, Alkhaldi TM, et al. Association between race/ethnicity and survival of melanoma patients in the United States over 3 decades: a secondary analysis of SEER data. Medicine (Baltimore). 2016;95(17):e3315.
33. Zheng YJ, Ho C, Lazar A, Ortiz-Urda S. Poor melanoma outcomes and survival in Asian Americans and Pacific Islanders. J Am Acad Dermatol. 2020; https://doi.org/10.1016/j.jaad.2020.08.086.
34. Hutcheson ACS, McGowan JW, Maize JC, Cook J. Multiple primary acral melanomas in African-Americans: a case series and review of the literature. Dermatologic Surg. 2007;33(1):1–10.
35. Gloster HM, Neal K. Skin cancer in skin of color. J Am Acad Dermatol. 2006;55(5):741–60. quiz 761–4
36. Cormier JN, Xing Y, Ding M, Lee JE, Mansfield PF, Gershenwald JE, et al. Ethnic differences among patients with cutaneous melanoma. Arch Intern Med. 2006;166(17):1907–14.
37. Byrd-Miles K, Toombs EL, Peck GL. Skin cancer in individuals of African, Asian, Latin-American, and American-Indian descent: differences in incidence, clinical presentation, and survival compared to Caucasians. J Drugs Dermatol. 2007;6(1):10–6.
38. Bergfelt L, Newell GR, Sider JG, Kripke ML. Incidence and anatomic distribution of cutaneous melanoma among United States Hispanics. J Surg Oncol. 1989;40(4):222–6.
39. Lv J, Dai B, Kong Y, Shen X, Kong J. Acral melanoma in Chinese: a Clinicopathological and prognostic study of 142 cases. Sci Rep. 2016;22(6):31432.
40. Lodder JV, Simson W, Becker PJ. Malignant melanoma of the skin in black South Africans: a 15-year experience. S Afr J Surg. 2010;48(3):76–9.
41. Halder RM, Bridgeman-Shah S. Skin cancer in African Americans. Cancer. 1995;75(S2): 667–73.

42. Cockburn MG, Zadnick J, Deapen D. Developing epidemic of melanoma in the Hispanic population of California. Cancer. 2006;106(5):1162–8.
43. Kuchelmeister C, Schaumburg-Lever G, Garbe C. Acral cutaneous melanoma in Caucasians: clinical features, histopathology and prognosis in 112 patients. Br J Dermatol. 2000;143(2):275–80.
44. O'Hanlon L. Invasive melanoma on the rise in Californian Hispanics. Lancet Oncol. 2006;7(3):199.
45. Hu S, Parker DF, Thomas AG, Kirsner RS. Advanced presentation of melanoma in African Americans: the Miami-Dade County experience. J Am Acad Dermatol. 2004;51(6):1031–2.
46. Pipitone M, Robinson JK, Camara C, Chittineni B, Fisher SG. Skin cancer awareness in suburban employees: a Hispanic perspective. J Am Acad Dermatol. 2002;47(1):118–23.
47. Rosenberg HM, Maurer JD, Sorlie PD, Johnson NJ, MacDorman MF, Hoyert DL, et al. Quality of death rates by race and Hispanic origin: a summary of current research, 1999. Vital Health Stat 2. 1999;128:1–13.
48. Saraiya M, Hall HI, Thompson T, Hartman A, Glanz K, Rimer B, et al. Skin cancer screening among U.S. adults from 1992, 1998, and 2000 National Health Interview Surveys. Prev Med. 2004;39(2):308–14.
49. Freeman HP. Poverty, culture, and social injustice: determinants of cancer disparities. CA Cancer J Clin. 2004;54(2):72–7.
50. Margolis ML, Christie JD, Silvestri GA, Kaiser L, Santiago S, Hansen-Flaschen J. Racial differences pertaining to a belief about lung cancer surgery: results of a multicenter survey. Ann Intern Med. 2003;139(7):558–63.
51. Ward E, Jemal A, Cokkinides V, Singh GK, Cardinez C, Ghafoor A, et al. Cancer disparities by race/ethnicity and socioeconomic status. CA Cancer J Clin. 2004;54(2):78–93.
52. Jemal A, Murray T, Ward E, Samuels A, Tiwari RC, Ghafoor A, et al. Cancer statistics, 2005. CA Cancer J Clin. 2005;55(1):10–30.
53. Pichon LC, Corral I, Landrine H, Mayer JA, Adams-Simms D. Perceived skin cancer risk and sunscreen use among African American adults. J Health Psychol. 2010;15(8):1181–9.
54. U.S. Cancer Statistics Working Group. U.S. Cancer Statistics Data Visualizations Tool, based on 2019 submission data (1999–2017): U.S. Department of Health and Human Services, Centers for Disease Control and Prevention and National Cancer Institute; [Internet]. [cited 2020 Sep 24]. www.cdc.gov/cancer/dataviz, released in June 2020.
55. Byrd KM, Wilson DC, Hoyler SS, Peck GL. Advanced presentation of melanoma in African Americans. J Am Acad Dermatol. 2004;50(1):21–4. https://doi.org/10.1016/S0190-9622(0 3)02091-7.

Melanoma Risk with Immunomodulators

Introduction

A functioning immune system is important for the prevention of malignancies. "Cancer immunoediting" describes three main processes: elimination, equilibrium, and escape. Elimination is the phase involving detection and elimination of tumor cells by the innate immune system. If elimination is unsuccessful, there is selection for tumor cells that can better resist the immune system in the equilibrium phase. In the escape process, tumor cells escape this control through genetic or epigenetic changes, leading to clinically observable malignant disease [1].

A few observations suggest that melanoma is an immunogenic tumor. Primary melanomas often exhibit strong lymphocytic infiltration inducing partial or complete regression. The development of vitiligo as an immune process is a marker of improved prognosis in melanoma patients [2]. Furthermore, immunotherapy has been used for the past decade with remarkable long-term results [3, 4]. These observations lead to the question of whether immunosuppressive or immunomodulating drugs affect the balance between the immune system and melanoma. This chapter summarizes the use of immunomodulating agents and whether their use requires consideration for more dermatological follow-up in monitoring for melanoma.

Melanoma Development in Immunosuppressed Patients

In organ transplant recipients (OTRs), there is an increased risk for non-melanoma skin cancers, but it remains controversial whether there is an increased risk of melanoma [5]. Some large population studies found no increased risk for melanoma in immunosuppressed patients, while others show a 2.1- to eight-fold higher incidence than in the general population [6]. Given the multidrug nature of immunosuppression therapy, studies typically cannot attribute any increased melanoma risk to a specific drug.

Inflammatory conditions such as rheumatoid arthritis (RA), psoriasis, and inflammatory bowel disease also require significant immunosuppressive therapy. A meta-analysis of malignancies in rheumatoid arthritis patients found an increased risk of melanoma with an increased standardized incidence ratio (SIR) of 1.23 (95% CI 1.01–1.49) but noted that study results were mixed [7]. Studies examining melanoma risk in patients with psoriasis or inflammatory bowel disease are also conflicting [8, 9].

Increased Melanoma Risk

The calcineurin inhibitors, cyclosporine and tacrolimus, decrease T-cell-mediated immunity by inhibiting the production of interleukin-2 (IL-2) and increasing the production of TGF-β1 [10–12]. A retrospective case-control study found that among renal transplant recipients, cyclosporine use was associated with increased risk of developing melanoma compared to patients who did not use cyclosporine, with a hazard ratio of 1.93 (95% CI 1.24–2.99; $P = 0.004$) [13]. A number of case reports also describe patients who developed melanoma after being treated with cyclosporine monotherapy [14–16]. However, in a post-marketing surveillance study for cyclosporine, only one case of melanoma was reported in more than 10,000 patients [17]. No studies report an increased risk of melanoma in patients treated with tacrolimus. Large meta-analyses have not found any correlation between the use of topical tacrolimus and the development of melanoma [18, 19].

The mammalian target of rapamycin (mTOR) is inhibited by the drugs sirolimus, temsirolimus, and everolimus. These drugs halt the progression from the G1 to S phase of the cell cycle, suppressing T-cell proliferation. However, through a similar mechanism, mTOR inhibitors also have anti-oncogenic effects [20, 21]. Two studies suggest that switching from calcineurin inhibitors to sirolimus may increase antitumoral effects among kidney transplant recipients with previous squamous cell carcinoma [22, 23]. However, one retrospective case-control study found that among renal transplant patients, use of sirolimus was associated with a hazard ratio of 1.54 (95% CI 1.22–1.94; $P < 0.001$) of developing melanoma compared to those who did not use sirolimus [13]. No association between either temsirolimus or everolimus and skin cancers have been found and both have been tried unsuccessfully as a treatment for melanoma [21, 24, 25].

Natalizumab is a monoclonal antibody targeting the alpha-4 subunit of integrin molecules, blocking leukocyte adhesion and transmigration. Case reports have described patients who developed melanoma during therapy with natalizumab [26–29]. Importantly, a study examining the FDA Adverse Events Reporting System across 10 years found 205 melanoma cases after natalizumab therapy for multiple sclerosis, which corresponded to a proportional reporting ratio of 2.42 (95% CI 2.10–2.8) [30]. Patients treated with natalizumab also appear to be diagnosed of melanoma at a younger median age of 45 [30]. These findings suggest that natalizumab exposure may be a risk factor for melanoma.

No Increased Melanoma Risk

The inhibitors of cytokines IL-6, IL-12, and IL-23 suppress the immune system but are not associated with increased melanoma risk. IL-6 is a strong inflammatory mediator with functions from reducing T-cell apoptosis to promoting tumorigenesis [31]. Tocilizumab is an IL-6 receptor antagonist that is being tested in clinical trials for treating advanced melanoma [32]. Large studies found no increased risk for malignancies compared to placebo [33–35]. IL-12 is involved in the induction of the innate immune system, promoting a Th1 response and elimination of cancer cells [36]. IL-23, on the other hand, is associated with a Th17 response, which decreases CD8+ T-cell infiltration and increases angiogenesis [37, 38]. Ustekinumab prevents binding of both IL-12 and IL-23, and clinical trials have not identified an increased risk of malignancy [39–41].

Cyclophosphamide is an alkylating chemotherapeutic and immunosuppressive agent whose metabolite crosslinks DNA, interfering with DNA synthesis. Although there may be an increased risk of urinary bladder cancer and acute myeloid leukemia, there does not appear to be an increased risk of melanoma [42–46].

Mycophenolate mofetil is a prodrug of mycophenolic acid, which inhibits inosine monophosphate dehydrogenase, a key enzyme in the de novo guanosine nucleotide synthesis, and primarily affects lymphocytes [47]. One large retrospective study demonstrated that patients treated with mycophenolate mofetil do not have an increased risk of malignancies compared to patients treated with other immunosuppression regimens [48]. Other studies describe melanoma in organ transplant patients, but do not have comparisons to controls to quantify any risk from mycophenolate mofetil [49–51].

Glucocorticoids are used to treat many inflammatory, allergic, immunologic, and malignant disorders for its effect on suppressing the innate and adaptive immune system. In two large case-control studies, systemic treatment with glucocorticoids was associated with an increased risk of non-melanoma skin cancer, but not an increased risk of melanoma [52, 53]. One case-control study demonstrated a protective effect of glucocorticoids on melanoma risk with odds ratio of 0.39 (95% CI: 0.2–0.74) [54].

Inconclusive Melanoma Risk

Some immunomodulator drugs have a debatable risk for melanoma with limited available evidence. Methotrexate blocks dihydrofolate reductase and thymidylate synthetase resulting in decreased nucleotide synthesis. A retrospective study evaluating the use of methotrexate for treating patients with rheumatoid arthritis found a threefold increased risk of developing melanoma compared to the general population with a standardized incidence ratio of 3.0 (95% CI: 1.2–6.2) [55]. Another retrospective study found a small but significant increased risk of 5-year risk of melanoma in patients treated with methotrexate (0.48%, 95% CI: 0.43–0.53%) compared to patients never treated with methotrexate (0.41%, 95% CI 0.39–0.43)

[56]. An evaluation of six studies in a meta-analysis found no significant increase in melanoma risk [57].

Tumor necrosis factor alpha (TNFα) inhibitors such as etanercept, infliximab, adalimumab, certolizumab pegol, and golimumab block the cytokine's pro-inflammatory and antitumor effects. Multiple meta-analyses have not found any association between TNFα inhibitors and cancer risk. However, one meta-analysis of TNFα inhibitor use for treating patients with rheumatoid arthritis found a statistically significant increased risk of melanoma with a pooled standardized incidence ratio of 1.7 (95% CI: 0.8–2.3) [58]. Observational studies have found a nonsignificant trend toward increased melanoma risk with infliximab (OR = 2.6, 95% CI: 1.0–6.7) and etanercept (OR = 2.4, 95% CI: 1.0–5.8), but not with adalimumab [59].

Azathioprine is another antimetabolite that antagonizes nucleotide synthesis, which limits lymphocyte proliferation. A meta-analysis of patients treated with thiopurines for inflammatory bowel disease found an increased risk of non-melanoma skin cancer but no statistically significantly increased melanoma risk (RR = 1.22, 95% CI 0.90–1.65, $P = 0.206$) [60].

Risk of Melanoma Progression or Recurrence

Generally, patients with a diagnosis of early melanoma are considered cured and discharged from close follow-up after 5 to 10 years. However, up to 6.9% of melanoma patients experience a late recurrence that can occur even 10 years after the initial diagnosis [61, 62]. Retrospective studies have investigated the risk of disease progression or recurrence after transplantation in patients with a history of melanoma. One retrospective study reported a melanoma recurrence rate of 19% (6 out of 31 patients) after solid organ transplantation [63]. Several other studies of patients with a history of melanoma before transplantation found no increased risk for recurrence or progression [6, 64–66]. Therefore, a history of melanoma should not be a contraindication to receiving solid organ transplantation.

Melanoma Prognosis during Immunosuppressant Treatment

Patients who develop melanoma after organ transplantation and require immunomodulating therapy may require closer follow-up depending on their tumor characteristics. Patients with thicker melanoma tumors (>1.51 mm Breslow depth or Clark III/IV) on immunomodulating therapy may have worse survival compared to AJCC control patients with thick melanomas (HR = 11.49, 95% CI 3.59–36.82) [65]. However, no increased risk from immunomodulating therapy was found for patients with thinner tumors [64]. One case-control study of melanoma patients with concomitant immunosuppressive therapy compared to matched-control patients not receiving immunologic treatment found similar relapse rates but were more likely to die from melanoma (42% in immunosuppressive treatment vs. 23% in controls,

$p = 0.01$) [67]. Therefore, there may be greater imperative to identify melanoma lesions early in patients on immunosuppressive treatment.

Conclusion

It may be prudent to offer more routine dermatologic examinations for patients treated with drugs associated with melanoma development. There appears to be epidemiologic evidence that some immunosuppressive drugs, including cyclosporine, natalizumab, and sirolimus, are associated with melanoma. A full assessment of melanoma risk should be considered alongside traditional risk factors for melanoma, such as fair skin, ultraviolet exposure, and personal/family history. For patients treated on drugs where the current level of evidence is unclear, increased follow-up may also be considered.

References

1. Dunn GP, Bruce AT, Ikeda H, Old LJ, Schreiber RD. Cancer immunoediting: from immunosurveillance to tumor escape. Nat Immunol. 2002;3(11):991–8.
2. Quaglino P, Marenco F, Osella-Abate S, Bernengo MG. Vitiligo is an independent favourable prognostic factor in stage III and IV metastatic melanoma patients: results from a single-institution hospital-based observational cohort study. Ann Oncol. 2010;21(2):409–14.
3. Atkins MB, Kunkel L, Sznol M, Rosenberg SA. High-dose recombinant interleukin-2 therapy in patients with metastatic melanoma: long-term survival update. Cancer J Sci Am. 2000;6(Suppl 1):S11–4.
4. Di Giacomo AM, Calabrò L, Danielli R, Fonsatti E, Bertocci E, Pesce I, et al. Long-term survival and immunological parameters in metastatic melanoma patients who responded to ipilimumab 10 mg/kg within an expanded access programme. Cancer Immunol Immunother. 2013;62(6):1021–8.
5. Madan V, Lear JT, Szeimies RM. Non-melanoma skin cancer. Lancet. 2010;375(9715):673–85.
6. Kubica AW, Brewer JD. Melanoma in immunosuppressed patients. Mayo Clin Proc Mayo Clin. 2012;87(10):991–1003.
7. Simon TA, Thompson A, Gandhi KK, Hochberg MC, Suissa S. Incidence of malignancy in adult patients with rheumatoid arthritis: a meta-analysis. Arthritis Res Ther. 2015;17:212.
8. Geller S, Xu H, Lebwohl M, Nardone B, Lacouture ME, Kheterpal M. Malignancy risk and recurrence with psoriasis and its treatments: a concise update. Am J Clin Dermatol. 2018;19(3):363–75.
9. Greuter T, Vavricka S, König AO, Beaugerie L, Scharl M, Swiss IBDnet, an official working group of the Swiss Society of Gastroenterology. Malignancies in inflammatory bowel disease. Digestion. 2020;101(Suppl 1):136–45.
10. Prashar Y, Khanna A, Sehajpal P, Sharma VK, Suthanthiran M. Stimulation of transforming growth factor-beta 1 transcription by cyclosporine. FEBS Lett. 1995;358(2):109–12.
11. Maluccio M, Sharma V, Lagman M, Vyas S, Yang H, Li B, et al. Tacrolimus enhances transforming growth factor-beta1 expression and promotes tumor progression. Transplantation. 2003;76(3):597–602.
12. Teicher BA. Malignant cells, directors of the malignant process: role of transforming growth factor-beta. Cancer Metastasis Rev. 2001;20(1–2):133–43.
13. Ascha M, Ascha MS, Tanenbaum J, Bordeaux JS. Risk factors for melanoma in renal transplant recipients. JAMA Dermatol. 2017;153(11):1130–6.

14. Mérot Y, Miescher PA, Balsiger F, Magnenat P, Frenk E. Cutaneous malignant melanomas occurring under cyclosporin a therapy: a report of two cases. Br J Dermatol. 1990;123(2):237–9.
15. Gallagher MP, Kelly PJ, Jardine M, Perkovic V, Cass A, Craig JC, et al. Long-term cancer risk of immunosuppressive regimens after kidney transplantation. J Am Soc Nephrol. 2010;21(5):852–8.
16. Tjon ASW, Sint Nicolaas J, Kwekkeboom J, de Man RA, Kazemier G, Tilanus HW, et al. Increased incidence of early de novo cancer in liver graft recipients treated with cyclosporine: an association with C2 monitoring and recipient age. Liver Transpl. 2010;16(7):837–46.
17. Arellano F, Krupp PF. Cutaneous malignant melanoma occurring after cyclosporin A therapy. Br J Dermatol. 1991;124(6):611.
18. Hui RL, Lide W, Chan J, Schottinger J, Yoshinaga M, Millares M. Association between exposure to topical tacrolimus or pimecrolimus and cancers. Ann Pharmacother. 2009;43(12):1956–63.
19. Tennis P, Gelfand JM, Rothman KJ. Evaluation of cancer risk related to atopic dermatitis and use of topical calcineurin inhibitors. Br J Dermatol. 2011;165(3):465–73.
20. de Fijter JW. Cancer and mTOR inhibitors in transplant recipients. Transplantation. 2017;101(1):45–55.
21. Holdaas H, De Simone P, Zuckermann A. Everolimus and malignancy after solid organ transplantation: a clinical update. J Transplant [Internet]. 2016; [cited 2021 May 3];2016. Available from: https://www.ncbi.nlm.nih.gov/pmc/articles/PMC5078653/
22. Euvrard S, Morelon E, Rostaing L, Goffin E, Brocard A, Tromme I, et al. Sirolimus and secondary skin-cancer prevention in kidney transplantation. N Engl J Med. 2012;367(4):329–39.
23. Campbell SB, Walker R, Tai SS, Jiang Q, Russ GR. Randomized controlled trial of sirolimus for renal transplant recipients at high risk for nonmelanoma skin cancer. Am J Transplant. 2012;12(5):1146–56.
24. Hauke RJ, Infante JR, Rubin MS, Shih KC, Arrowsmith ER, Hainsworth JD. Everolimus in combination with paclitaxel and carboplatin in patients with metastatic melanoma: a phase II trial of the Sarah Cannon Research Institute Oncology Research Consortium. Melanoma Res. 2013;23(6):468–73.
25. Velho TR. Metastatic melanoma—a review of current and future drugs. Drugs Context [Internet]. 2012; Nov 19 [cited 2021 Jun 1];2012. Available from: https://www.ncbi.nlm.nih.gov/pmc/articles/PMC3885142/
26. Mullen JT, Vartanian TK, Atkins MB. Melanoma complicating treatment with natalizumab for multiple sclerosis. N Engl J Med. 2008;358(6):647–8.
27. Bergamaschi R, Montomoli C. Melanoma in multiple sclerosis treated with natalizumab: causal association or coincidence? Mult Scler. 2009;15(12):1532–3.
28. Vavricka BMP, Baumberger P, Russmann S, Kullak-Ublick GA. Diagnosis of melanoma under concomitant natalizumab therapy. Mult Scler. 2011;17(2):255–6.
29. Laroni A, Bedognetti M, Uccelli A, Capello E, Mancardi GL. Association of melanoma and natalizumab therapy in the Italian MS population: a second case report. Neurol Sci. 2011;32(1):181–2.
30. Kelm RC, Hagstrom EL, Mathieu RJ, Orrell KA, Serrano L, Mueller KA, et al. Melanoma subsequent to natalizumab exposure: a report from the RADAR (research on adverse drug events and reports) program. J Am Acad Dermatol. 2019;80(3):820–1.
31. Kumari N, Dwarakanath BS, Das A, Bhatt AN. Role of interleukin-6 in cancer progression and therapeutic resistance. Tumour Biol. 2016;37(9):11553–72.
32. NYU Langone Health. A phase II study of the interleukin-6 receptor inhibitor tocilizumab in combination with ipilimumab and nivolumab in patients with unresectable stage III or stage IV melanoma [Internet]. clinicaltrials.gov; 2021 May [cited 2021 May 31]. Report No.: NCT03999749. Available from: https://clinicaltrials.gov/ct2/show/NCT03999749
33. Nishimoto N. Interleukin-6 as a therapeutic target in candidate inflammatory diseases. Clin Pharmacol Ther. 2010;87(4):483–7.
34. Patel AM, Moreland LW. Interleukin-6 inhibition for treatment of rheumatoid arthritis: a review of tocilizumab therapy. Drug Des Devel Ther. 2010;4:263–78.

35. Bannwarth B, Richez C. Clinical safety of tocilizumab in rheumatoid arthritis. Expert Opin Drug Saf. 2011;10(1):123–31.
36. Yan J, Smyth MJ, Teng MWL. Interleukin (IL)-12 and IL-23 and their conflicting roles in cancer. Cold Spring Harb Perspect Biol. 2018;10(7):a028530.
37. Langowski JL, Zhang X, Wu L, Mattson JD, Chen T, Smith K, et al. IL-23 promotes tumour incidence and growth. Nature. 2006;442(7101):461–5.
38. Lyakh L, Trinchieri G, Provezza L, Carra G, Gerosa F. Regulation of interleukin-12/interleukin-23 production and the T-helper 17 response in humans. Immunol Rev. 2008;226:112–31.
39. Quatresooz P, Hermanns-Lê T, Piérard GE, Humbert P, Delvenne P, Piérard-Franchimont C. Ustekinumab in psoriasis immunopathology with emphasis on the Th17-IL23 axis: a primer. J Biomed Biotechnol. 2012;2012:147413.
40. Gordon KB, Papp KA, Langley RG, Ho V, Kimball AB, Guzzo C, et al. Long-term safety experience of ustekinumab in patients with moderate to severe psoriasis (part II of II): results from analyses of infections and malignancy from pooled phase II and III clinical trials. J Am Acad Dermatol. 2012;66(5):742–51.
41. Panaccione R, Danese S, Sandborn WJ, O'Brien CD, Zhou Y, Zhang H, et al. Ustekinumab is effective and safe for ulcerative colitis through 2 years of maintenance therapy. Aliment Pharmacol Ther. 2020;52(11–12):1658–75.
42. Baker GL, Kahl LE, Zee BC, Stolzer BL, Agarwal AK, Medsger TAJ. Malignancy following treatment of rheumatoid arthritis with cyclophosphamide. Long-term case-control follow-up study. Am J Med. 1987;83(1):1–9.
43. Bernatsky S, Ramsey-Goldman R, Clarke AE. Malignancies and cyclophosphamide exposure in Wegener's granulomatosis. J Rheumatol. 2008;35(1):11–3.
44. Faurschou M, Sorensen IJ, Mellemkjaer L, Loft AGR, Thomsen BS, Tvede N, et al. Malignancies in Wegener's granulomatosis: incidence and relation to cyclophosphamide therapy in a cohort of 293 patients. J Rheumatol. 2008;35(1):100–5.
45. Pedersen-Bjergaard J, Ersbøll J, Hansen VL, Sørensen BL, Christoffersen K, Hou-Jensen K, et al. Carcinoma of the urinary bladder after treatment with cyclophosphamide for non-Hodgkin's lymphoma. N Engl J Med. 1988;318(16):1028–32.
46. van den Brand JAJG, van Dijk PR, Hofstra JM, Wetzels JFM. Cancer risk after cyclophosphamide treatment in idiopathic membranous nephropathy. Clin J Am Soc Nephrol. 2014;9(6):1066–73.
47. Allison AC, Eugui EM. Mycophenolate mofetil and its mechanisms of action. Immunopharmacology. 2000;47(2–3):85–118.
48. Robson R, Cecka JM, Opelz G, Budde M, Sacks S. Prospective registry-based observational cohort study of the long-term risk of malignancies in renal transplant patients treated with mycophenolate mofetil. Am J Transplant. 2005;5(12):2954–60.
49. Cohen BE, Krivitskiy I, Bui S, Forrester K, Kahn J, Barbers R, et al. Comparison of skin cancer incidence in Caucasian and non-Caucasian liver vs. lung transplant recipients: a tale of two regimens. Clin Drug Investig. 2019;39(2):197–203.
50. Sodemann U, Bistrup C, Marckmann P. Cancer rates after kidney transplantation. Dan Med Bull. 2011;58(12):A4342.
51. Puza CJ, Cardones AR, Mosca PJ. Examining the incidence and presentation of melanoma in the cardiothoracic transplant population. JAMA Dermatol. 2018;154(5):589.
52. Sørensen HT, Mellemkjaer L, Nielsen GL, Baron JA, Olsen JH, Karagas MR. Skin cancers and non-hodgkin lymphoma among users of systemic glucocorticoids: a population-based cohort study. J Natl Cancer Inst. 2004;96(9):709–11.
53. Jensen AØ, Thomsen HF, Engebjerg MC, Olesen AB, Friis S, Karagas MR, et al. Use of oral glucocorticoids and risk of skin cancer and non-Hodgkin's lymphoma: a population-based case-control study. Br J Cancer. 2009;100(1):200–5.
54. Landi MT, Baccarelli A, Calista D, Fears TR, Landi G. Glucocorticoid use and melanoma risk. Int J Cancer. 2001;94(2):302–3.

55. Buchbinder R, Barber M, Heuzenroeder L, Wluka AE, Giles G, Hall S, et al. Incidence of melanoma and other malignancies among rheumatoid arthritis patients treated with methotrexate. Arthritis Rheum. 2008;59(6):794–9.
56. Polesie S, Gillstedt M, Sönnergren HH, Osmancevic A, Paoli J. Methotrexate treatment and risk for cutaneous malignant melanoma: a retrospective comparative registry-based cohort study. Br J Dermatol. 2017;176(6):1492–9.
57. Pouplard C, Brenaut E, Horreau C, Barnetche T, Misery L, Richard MA, et al. Risk of cancer in psoriasis: a systematic review and meta-analysis of epidemiological studies. J Eur Acad Dermatol Venereol. 2013;27(s3):36–46.
58. Olsen CM, Green AC. Risk of invasive melanoma in patients with rheumatoid arthritis treated with biologics: an updated meta-analysis. Ann Rheum Dis. 2018;77(8):e49.
59. Wolfe F, Michaud K. Biologic treatment of rheumatoid arthritis and the risk of malignancy: analyses from a large US observational study. Arthritis Rheum. 2007;56(9):2886–95.
60. Huang SZ, Liu ZC, Liao WX, Wei JX, Huang XW, Yang C, et al. Risk of skin cancers in thiopurines-treated and thiopurines-untreated patients with inflammatory bowel disease: a systematic review and meta-analysis. J Gastroenterol Hepatol. 2019;34(3):507–16.
61. Pescarini E, Spanikova G, Mbaidjol Z, De Antoni E, Vindigni V, Bassetto F. Late metastatic melanoma after 25 years: a case report and a brief literature review. Case Rep Surg. 2020;2020:e2938236.
62. Faries MB, Steen S, Ye X, Sim M, Morton DL. Late recurrence in melanoma: clinical implications of lost dormancy. J Am Coll Surg. 2013;217(1):27–34.
63. Penn I. Malignant melanoma in organ allograft recipients. Transplantation. 1996;61(2):274–8.
64. Brewer JD, Christenson LJ, Weaver AL, Dapprich DC, Weenig RH, Lim KK, et al. Malignant melanoma in solid transplant recipients: collection of database cases and comparison with surveillance, epidemiology, and end results data for outcome analysis. Arch Dermatol. 2011;147(7):790–6.
65. Matin RN, Mesher D, Proby CM, McGregor JM, Bouwes Bavinck JN, del Marmol V, et al. Melanoma in organ transplant recipients: clinicopathological features and outcome in 100 cases. Am J Transplant. 2008;8(9):1891–900.
66. Colegio OR, Proby CM, Bordeaux JS, McGregor JM, Melanoma Working Group of the International Transplant Skin Cancer Collaborative (ITSCC) & Skin Care in Organ Transplant Patients, Europe (SCOPE). Prognosis of pretransplant melanoma. Am J Transplant. 2009;9(4):862.
67. Frankenthaler A, Sullivan RJ, Wang W, Renzi S, Seery V, Lee MY, et al. Impact of concomitant immunosuppression on the presentation and prognosis of patients with melanoma. Melanoma Res. 2010;20(6):496–500.

Dermoscopy

Dermoscopy Background

Dermoscopy (also known as epiluminescence microscopy, dermatoscopy, and skin-surface microscopy) is a simple, noninvasive in vivo method to closely examine skin lesions [1, 2]. By visualizing morphological features not seen by the naked eye, dermoscopy links clinical dermatology with dermatopathology to allow one to distinguish melanoma from other melanocytic and nonmelanocytic pigmented skin lesions [3]. Its use increases diagnostic accuracy by 5–30% over clinical visual inspection alone, depending on the type of skin lesion and experience of the physician [4–6]. Dermoscopy in conjunction with total body photography can reduce the number of excisions required, with a 3:1 benign-malignant ratio of biopsy specimens, compared to 9:1 with just photography [7].

When identifying a lesion, it is helpful to first determine whether it is melanocytic or nonmelanocytic. If it is unclear, then it should be treated as if it is a melanocytic lesion by default [8]. After classifying lesions in this way, we can begin looking for more characteristic features to diagnose the lesion [8]. In this chapter we will describe general dermoscopic features of melanocytic lesions, discuss common examples of nonmelanocytic lesions, and then present classifications for melanocytic lesions (Fig. 15.1).

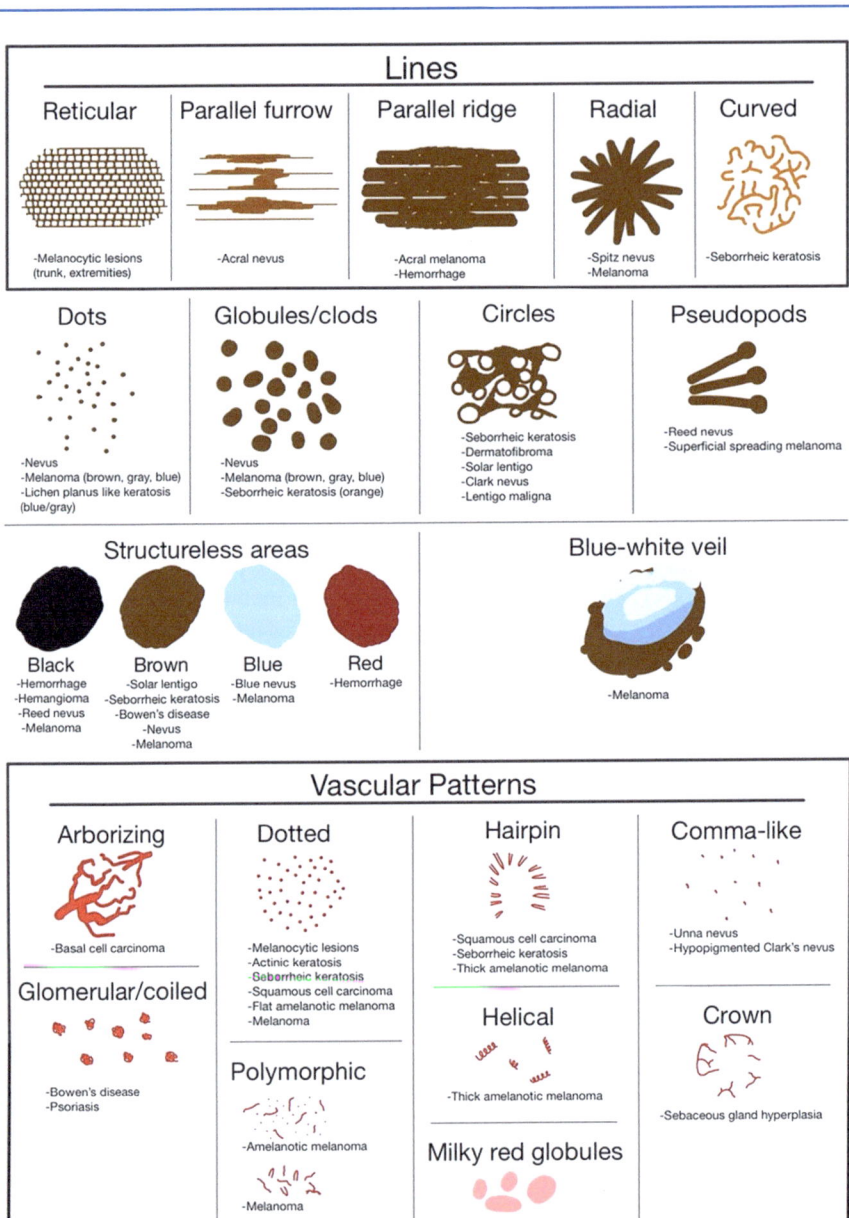

Fig. 15.1 Dermoscopic features

Features of Melanocytic Lesions

The Tyndall effect causes the color of melanin in lesions to depend on the depth of the pigment: black in the stratum corneum and upper epidermis, brown in the lower epidermis or dermal-epidermal junction, and blue gray in the dermis [9]. The pigment is distributed in varying patterns depending on its location on the body.

On the trunk or extremities, the distribution of pigment forms a pigment network, which is usually reticular (like a honeycomb or a net). This pattern exists because of the skin microanatomy, with greater overlap of pigmented cells lining the rete ridges from a superficial view [10]. In contrast, there is less overlap of pigmented cells over the dermal papillae, leading to the appearance of clear areas [10].

The head and neck regions have thinner skin and a relatively flat dermal-epidermal junction, so a typical pigment network is not seen here. However, appendageal openings such as hair follicles and sebaceous glands cause interruptions in the pigment distribution. This results in a pseudonetwork and is typically seen in melanocytic lesions but can also be seen in nonmelanocytic lesions [11, 12].

The acral surfaces of the palms and soles also do not have pronounced dermal papillae and rete ridges, but instead have furrows and ridges that form the lines and curves on these surfaces [13]. The furrows (also called fissures) are the sulci and, if pigmented, lead to the appearance of thin lines. The ridges are the gyri and, if pigmented, appear as broader lines with interruptions at the openings of sweat ducts. As we will discuss later, assessing the risk of acral melanocytic lesions depends on identifying whether the pigment is either in the furrows or in the ridges.

Sometimes melanin pigment might not be fully distributed, and this leads to the appearance of round or ovoid areas of pigment called dots (<0.1 mm) or globules (>0.1 mm). They represent nests of melanocytes, clumps of melanin, and/or melanophages at any level from the epidermis to the dermis [14, 15]. Uniform globules that are close to neighboring globules and form angulated borders are described to have a cobblestone pattern [8].

Pigment may also be distributed to form radial lines, which seem to have a center in the lesion from which pigment lines appear to radiate. Occasionally, the outer end of these lines may have a bulbous tip, forming a pseudopod. The term "streaks" encompasses both radial streaming and pseudopods. Symmetrical distribution of streaks around a lesion favors a diagnosis of Reed nevus (a type of Spitz nevus), whereas asymmetrical distribution favors superficial spreading melanoma [16]. Streaks represent lesions with rapid horizontal growth, with pseudopods having a high specificity for melanoma [17].

The pigment may also be homogeneously diffuse across a broad area without any of the dermoscopic features described above. A blue-white veil is an irregular, confluent blue-white structureless area that occupies less than the entire lesion. This feature has a 51% sensitivity and 97% specificity and represents pigment deposition in the superficial dermis with contact orthokeratosis, leading to a clinically elevated part of the lesion [16, 18–20].

Nonmelanocytic Lesions

Lentigines are macules with increased melanin pigmentation that develop with age and are like freckles but do not fade in the absence of sun exposure [21]. It appears that in lentigines, melanocytes and their precursors respond to signals from photo-damaged skin in a process driven by keratinocytes and fibroblasts [22, 23]. Although they are associated with increased number of melanocytes and melanoblasts, the cells do not have elevated proliferation markers [24].

Ink Spot Lentigo

Clinically, the ink spot lentigo (also called reticulated black solar lentigo) appears as a dark brown or black macule with an irregular outline [25]. The dark color, irregular border, and uncommon nature may cause the lesion to appear suspicious; however, dermoscopy allows the benign features to be visualized. One may see a prominent reticulated pattern of pigment that may be irregularly disrupted [26]. The key to distinguishing an ink spot lentigo from other pigmented lesions is noticing that in between the reticulated pigment (tips of rete ridges), the pigmentation of the suprapapillary plates resembles that of surrounding skin.

Solar Lentigo

The solar lentigo is an irregular brown or tan macule that develops on sun-exposed skin [27]. Using dermoscopy, the solar lentigo has a fine reticular network with thinner lines and larger holes and ends abruptly at the periphery without fading [28]. Solar lentigines are considered precursor lesions of seborrheic keratosis and it may be possible to see comedo-like openings or milia-like cysts (discussed in the seborrheic keratosis section below), which suggest that the lesion is in the process of transformation [27]. Lentigo maligna is included in the differential diagnosis, and dermoscopy is required to differentiate the two. Two features that are specific for lentigo maligna are asymmetrical pigmentation around follicular openings and rhomboid structures [29] (Fig. 15.2).

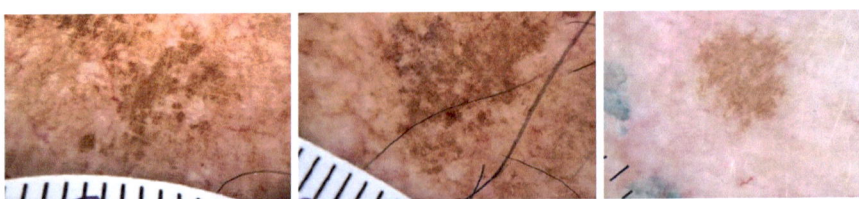

Fig. 15.2 Solar lentigo. Reticular network has large holes and ends abruptly at the periphery

Fig. 15.3 Seborrheic keratosis. Pigmented fissures, comedo-like openings, scale

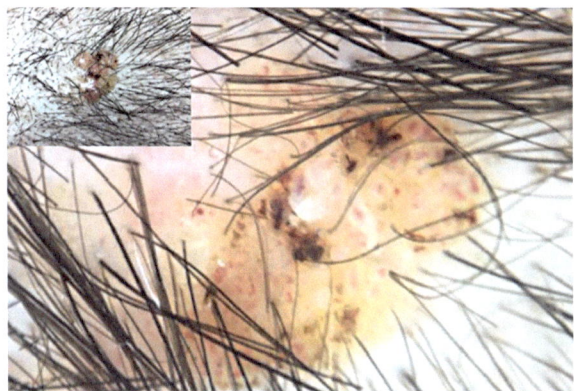

Seborrheic Keratosis

Seborrheic keratosis can be difficult to clinically distinguish from melanoma, especially when they are pigmented. It tends to have a scaly surface and the borders are sharply demarcated. Dermoscopy can reveal some very distinct features. One finding is the lack of a pigment network and instead, there may be pigmented fissures and lighter ridges that can be linear or branch irregularly [30]. This pattern may appear brain-like or cerebriform. Also visible may be milia-like cysts that are small bright white or yellow structures that correspond to intraepidermal keratin cysts, producing a "stars in the sky" appearance [31]. If the collection of keratin is open to the surface, as in keratotic invaginations (pseudohorn cysts), they form comedo-like openings that may be darkly pigmented and can be confused with dots/globules of melanocytic lesions [31]. A nonspecific finding that often appears in seborrheic keratosis are hairpin vessels with a surrounding hypopigmented halo [32] (Fig. 15.3).

Basal Cell Carcinoma

There are a few criteria to make the dermoscopic diagnosis of basal cell carcinoma. Firstly, there must not be a pigment network. One of the most sensitive and specific findings are the presence of arborizing blood vessels, which are branching telangiectasias. Although arborizing vessels are overwhelmingly found in basal cell carcinoma, they may also be found in other tumors including melanoma [33]. Although there is no pigment network, there is often some form of pigmented dots or globules with colors including black, brown, gray, blue, red, or white. One finding with high specificity but low sensitivity are pigmented spoke-wheel structures, which are focal areas of lines radial within the lesion. Erosions or ulcerations may be present and appear red or black from congealed blood forming a crust. Menzies et al. describe a model for diagnosing pigmented basal cell carcinoma with 93% sensitivity and 89% specificity, by having no pigment network and one or more of the following six features: large gray-blue ovoid nests, multiple gray-blue globules, maple

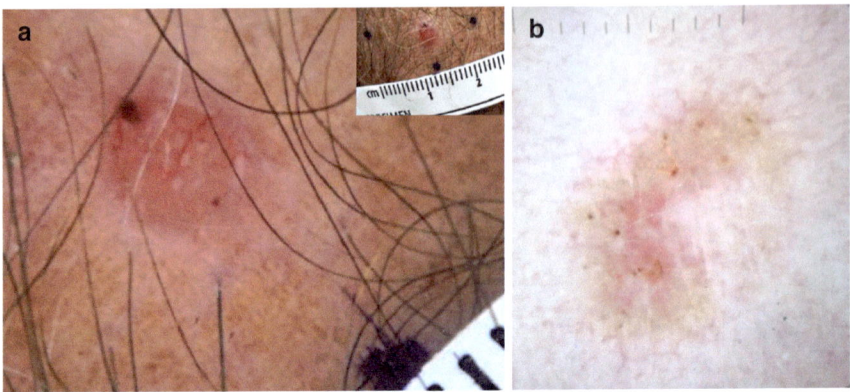

Fig. 15.4 Basal cell carcinoma. (**a**) Arborizing vessels, pink structureless area, gray-white peripherally. (**b**) Spoke-wheel structures, branching vessels; amelanotic melanoma is in the differential diagnosis

leaflike areas spoke wheel areas, ulceration, and arborizing telangiectasias [34] (Fig. 15.4).

Sebaceous Gland Hyperplasia

Sebaceous gland hyperplasia is a disorder of sebaceous gland that is common in middle age and older adults [35]. Characteristic of these lesions are white or yellow nodules near the center of the lesion [36]. When the ostium of the gland is visible, it appears as a small crater or umbilication at the center of the yellow nodules and is seen in 80% of sebaceous gland hyperplasias [37]. Crown vessels are vascular structures that surround the lesion and run toward the lesion center but never reach it, and one study found them in 5/6 sebaceous gland hyperplasias [38, 39].

Dermatofibroma

Also known as a fibrous histiocytoma, a dermatofibroma is a benign fibrohistiocytic mesenchymal growth. The hallmark feature of a dermatofibroma is a central homogeneous white region that appears like a scar. Unlike most other nonmelanocytic tumors, it is common to find a pigment network around the periphery of the lesion. With polarized dermoscopy, a characteristic feature is the visibility of blood vessels or a pink hue [40]. Some dermatofibromas appear atypical with features seen in regressive melanoma such as irregular pigment network and irregular dots/globules/blotches.

Vascular Lesions

Vascular lesions such as hemangiomas are sharply demarcated round or oval lesions. They present with different shades of red or blue and can be homogeneously black if the blood is thrombosed. Hemangiomas consist of lacunae or lagoons divided by white fibrous septae. Since lacunae in hemangiomas can resemble the saccules of metastatic melanoma, and the areas of blue and white can resemble a blue-white veil, it can be difficult to distinguish from metastatic melanoma.

Squamous Cell Carcinoma

Squamous cell carcinoma is the second most common cutaneous malignancy after basal cell carcinoma [41]. Actinic keratosis, also called solar keratosis, are precancerous forms of squamous cell carcinoma and the progression rate is 0–0.075% per lesion-year but can be up to 0.53% in patients with a history of nonmelanoma skin cancer [42]. Dermoscopically, actinic keratoses are characterized by erythema-reticular vessels that surround follicular openings, with white round keratotic dots in the follicular openings [43]. Bowen disease, or in situ squamous cell carcinoma, is classically described to have dotted or glomerular vessels [43, 44]. An invasive squamous cell carcinoma may have hairpin vessels with a surrounding halo and areas of erosion/ulceration characterized by red-brown structures from hemorrhage [43]. The presence of white circles, which correspond to keratin within the follicular openings, has a specificity of 87% for squamous cell carcinoma or keratoacanthoma [45] (Fig. 15.5).

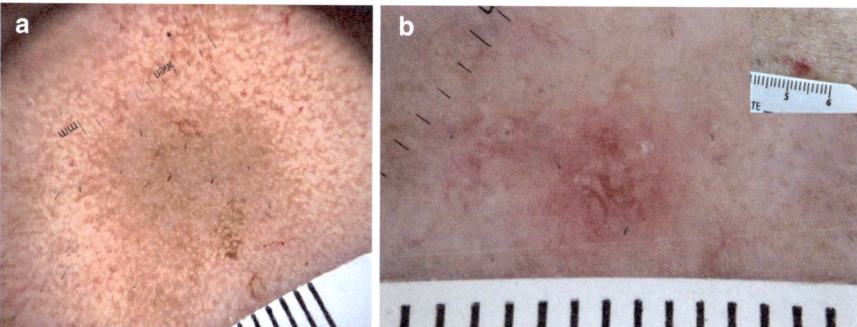

Fig. 15.5 Actinic keratosis. (**a**) Collision lesion of actinic keratosis and solar lentigo showing scattered reticular vessels that surround follicular openings. (**b**) Differential between actinic keratosis and Bowen disease in this lesion with coiled vessels

Stratifying Risk of Melanocytic Lesions

Just as there are the ABCDEs of grossly evaluating potential melanomas, a similar scheme of ABCD can be used in assessing with dermoscopy: asymmetry, border, color, and dermoscopic structures. Benign melanocytic lesions tend to have a large amount of symmetry with a regular pattern and a single uniform color. In contrast, malignant melanocytic lesions tend to have no symmetry with multiple irregular patterns and multiple colors. In thoroughly evaluating a lesion for risk, it can be helpful to have a checklist in mind with characteristics to look for. Table 15.1 depicts 3-point, 7-point, and Menzies method checklists.

Table 15.1 Dermoscopy checklists for melanoma

3-point checklist: ≥2 suggest high-risk lesion	7-point checklist: ≥3 suggest melanoma, *worth 2 points, otherwise 1 point	Menzies method: probable melanoma if both **negative features are true, and at least one positive feature
Asymmetrical color/structure		Cannot have symmetrical pattern** Cannot have just one color**
Irregular pigment network	Irregular pigment network*	Irregular pigment network
Blue/white color	Blue/white color* Polymorphous vascular patterns*	Blue/white color
	Irregular streaks	Irregular streaks Pseudopods
	Irregular dots/globules	Multiple brown dots Multiple blue-gray dots Peripheral black dots/globules
	Irregular blotches Regression	Scar-like depigmentation ≥5 colors

*Are worth two points in the 7-point checklist. All others are worth 1 point in the 7-point checklist.
**Are negative features. In Menzies method, both negative features and at least one positive feature is suggestive of melanoma.

Benign Melanocytic Lesions

Nevi of various types are likely benign if they have the general characteristics of a uniform pattern and one color, which can vary in shade.

Congenital Nevus

A wide range of melanocytic lesions can present congenitally including small (<1.5 cm), medium (1.5–19 cm), and giant (≥20 cm) [46]. Dermoscopic patterns include globular (most common in children), reticular (most common in adults), reticuloglobular, and homogeneous [47]. Other features include focal hypopigmentation and perifollicular hypopigmentation [48]. Congenital nevi may also be amelanotic and be pink, red, purple, or normal skin colored. Over the course of years, the lesion may grow in size and increase in hair density, but no other significant dermoscopic changes typically occur [49] (Fig. 15.6). A small but clinically significant proportion of congenital nevi undergo malignant transformation [50]. Large congenital nevi have an increased risk of malignant transformation on the order of 2.5 to 5% [51, 52].

Acquired Nevus

Acquired nevi begin appearing in the first decade of life and increase in number through adolescence [53]. Nevi that appear in childhood frequently have a globular pattern, while most nevi seen later in life will have a regular pigment network that fills the entire lesion. The evolution of the nevus is normal if the growth is dermoscopically organized, whereas disorganized growth with chaotic distribution suggests a malignant process [54]. At the periphery, the pigment network typically thins and fades in color (Fig. 15.7).

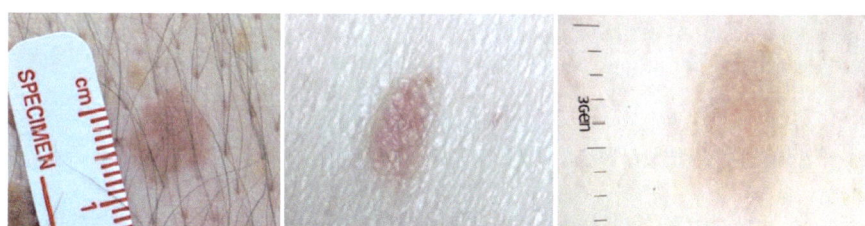

Fig. 15.6 Amelanotic nevus

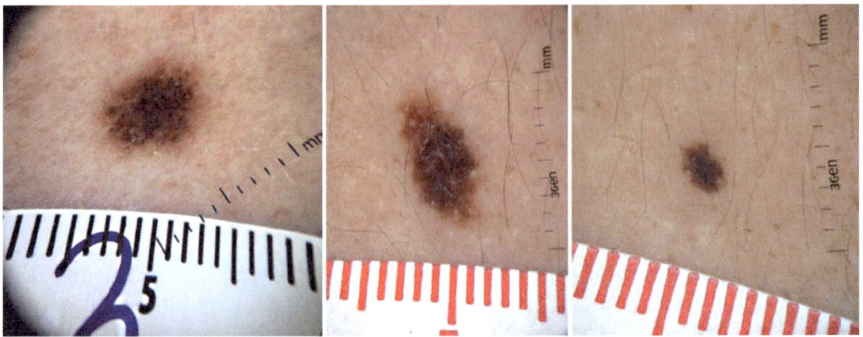

Fig. 15.7 Compound nevi. Nests of cells at the dermal-epidermal junction as well as within the dermis. Symmetrical pigment network fades at the periphery

Blue Nevus

A nevus that is blue, blue-gray, or blue-black produces this color because its melanin pigment is deeper in the dermis. They typically appear during childhood or adolescence and can be located on the head, neck, sacrum, or dorsum of the hands and feet [55]. Since this is below the dermal-epidermal junction, there is no pigment network and instead, the pigment is diffusely homogeneous across the lesion. It may be possible to see subtle blue globules in the homogeneous background. If there is regression, a white or gray color may also be seen. However, if there are structures such as a network, brown or black dots/globules, or vessels, the lesion may be a combined nevus or a melanoma [55].

Combined Nevus

A nevus may have both blue and brown color, representing the presence of pigment in the dermis and dermal-epidermal junction, respectively (Fig. 15.8). Although other combinations of these two colors exist, it is typically one color in the center and the other color around the border.

Unna and Miescher Nevi

Among intradermal nevi, two other classifications exist: Unna nevus and Miescher nevus. Most Miescher nevi are associated with the face and most Unna nevi are associated with the neck, trunk, and limbs [56]. Histopathologically, Miescher nevi melanocytes diffusely infiltrate the adventitial and deeper reticular dermis in a wedge-shaped pattern, whereas Unna nevi melanocytes are confined more superficially to the dermal adventitia and perifollicular dermis [56]. The Unna nevus may be indistinguishable from acrochordons, as soft, exophytic, smooth-surfaced or

Fig. 15.8 Combined nevus. Blue structureless center. Brown globules, reticular network

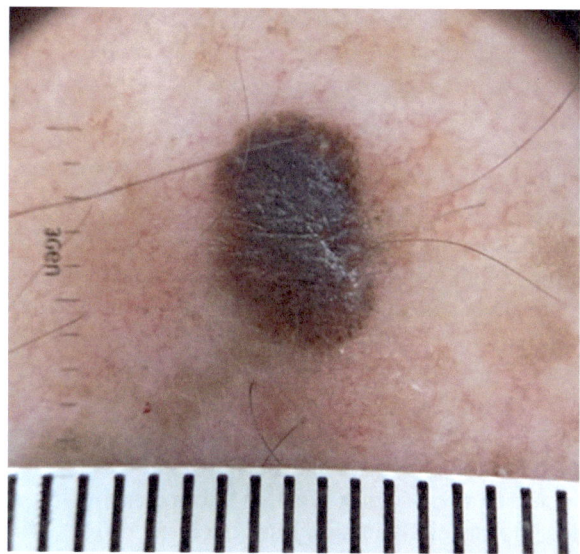

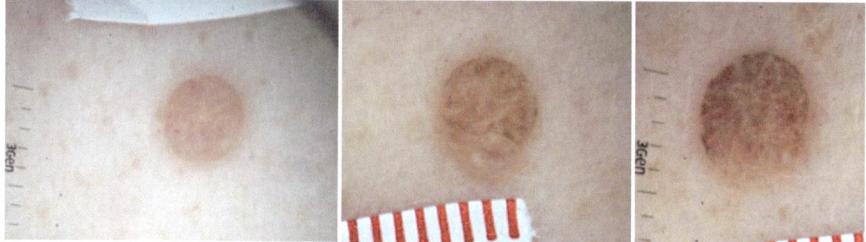

Fig. 15.9 Cellular/Unna nevus. Exophytic, uniform in color, and sharply demarcated

papillated, sessile or pedunculated, skin-colored or tan, uniform in color, sharply demarcated, and usually less than 1 cm in diameter [57] (Fig. 15.9). Dermoscopy of the Unna nevus may reveal a homogeneous and globular pattern, multifocal hypo/hyperpigmentation, and comma vessels [58].

Higher-Risk Melanocytic Lesions

Recurrent Nevus

In the location where a nevus was excised, the rare recurrence can lead to a lesion with several suspicious features that may include heterogeneous pigmentation, irregular network, or radial growth [59, 60]. The strongest clue to suggest a recurrent melanoma may be visualization of pigment that traverses the scar's edge [59]. Other features suggesting melanoma include chaotic or noncontinuous growth pattern [59]. Studies suggest that it may not be necessary to re-excise lesions that were incompletely removed if the initial pathology report indicates a benign or dysplastic nevus because of a very low rate of melanoma development [61–63].

Dysplastic Nevus

On the continuous spectrum of the appearance of melanocytic lesions from the common benign nevi to melanoma, dysplastic nevi lie somewhere in the middle with some atypical features (Fig. 15.10). These include lack of symmetry of color and structure and irregular dots/globules/blotches. Some features that are highly suggestive of melanoma and require a biopsy include a blue-white veil, polymorphous vessels, and radial streaks or pseudopods. It is argued that the term "dysplastic nevus" no longer be used since it is not associated with pathology different from benign-appearing nevi and only a minority carry mutations associated with an increased risk of transformation into melanoma [64–66]. This is supported by the fact that patients with dysplastic nevi that were biopsied and found to have positive histological margins do not develop melanoma [67, 68]. Despite this, there may be

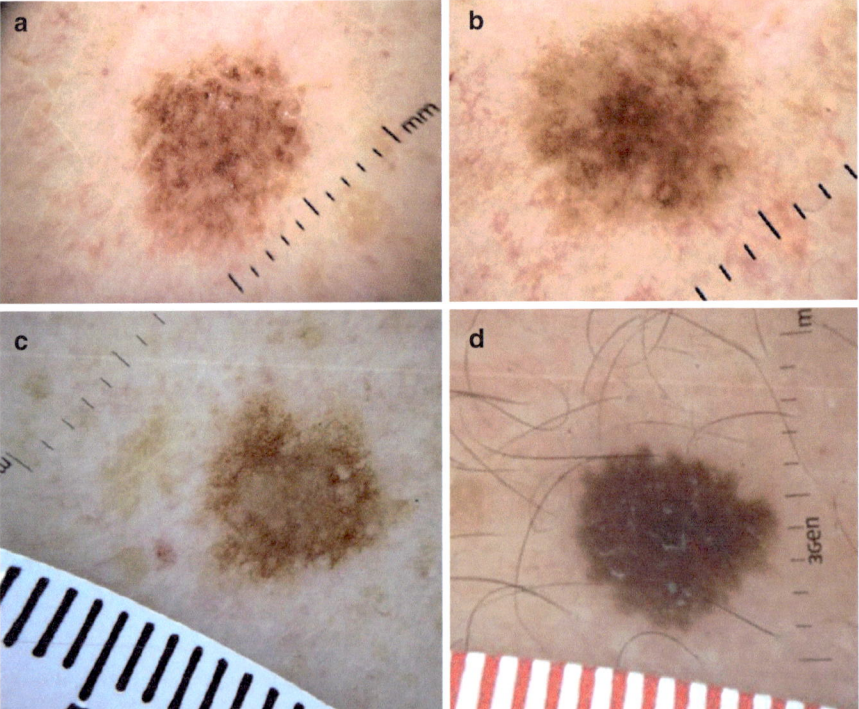

Fig. 15.10 Dysplastic nevi (**a**–**h**). Irregular pigmented network, gray dots, irregular borders. C, E, and F show signs of regression

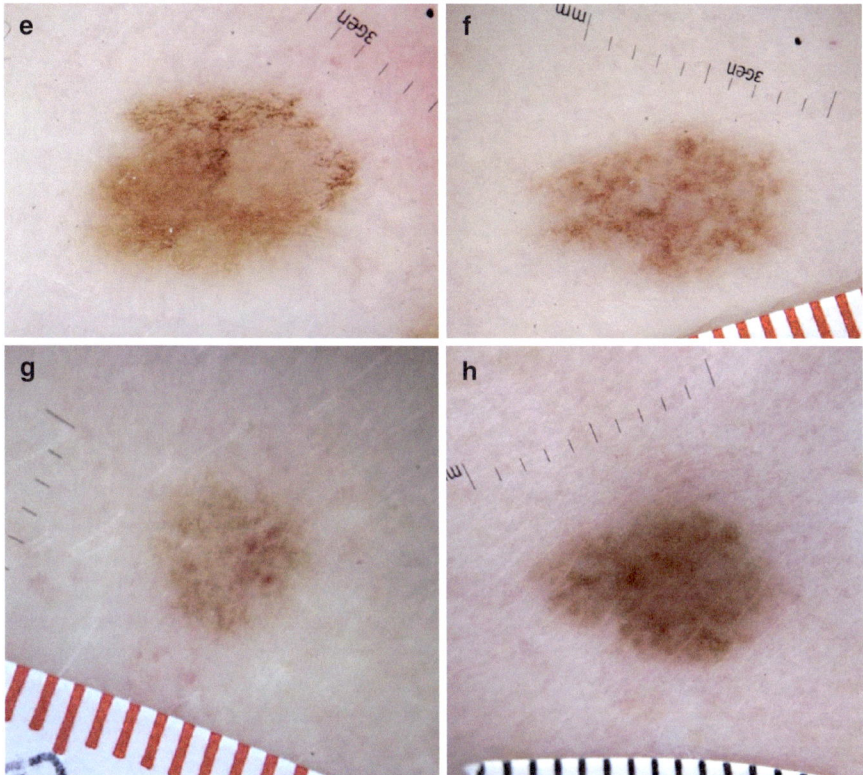

Fig. 15.10 (continued)

substantial overlap in the appearance of dysplastic nevi and in situ melanoma, so many physicians favor excision of these lesions [69].

Nevus Spilus

Also called speckled lentiginous nevus, a nevus spilus is a macule with a light brown background and numerous superimposed darker maculopapular speckles [70] (Fig. 15.11). They are relatively rare, as one study suggests at 2.8% of patients with melanoma risk factors who received total-body digital photography [71]. They present mostly within infancy but can occur at any age [72]. The concern is that melanoma may arise within the nevus spilus, though the rate is on the scale of 0.13% to 0.2% [70]. Although no standard exists, some authors suggest regular follow-up and self-examination [70, 72].

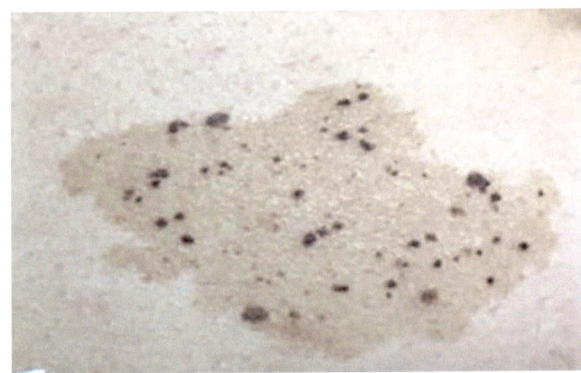

Fig. 15.11 Nevus spilus. Light brown background with darker brown globules of varying sizes

Spitz Nevus

Among several types of Spitz nevi, the two most common types are the starburst and the globular patterns [73]. The starburst pattern is named for the predominance of brown or black radial streaks with dots/globules at the periphery or pseudopods. The center of the lesion may be light or dark brown, black, or blue. The globular pattern Spitz nevus is filled with regular or irregular brown dots/globules and must also have reticular depigmentation [74]. In children, Spitz nevi are common and many are likely to involute [75]. In adults, however, Spitz nevus is rare and requires a histopathological diagnosis because it is highly likely that the lesion is a spitzoid melanoma.

Melanoma

Melanoma In Situ

Melanoma in situ refers to melanoma that remains within the epidermis and has not broken the basement membrane. Therefore, it would be a light to dark brown or black color and would not have characteristics of deeper melanomas such as regression or gray/blue color. Features to look for include asymmetry of color and structure, irregular pigment network, irregular dots/globules, and irregular dark blotches (Fig. 15.12).

Lentigo Maligna and Lentigo Maligna Melanoma

Lentigo maligna is a subtype of melanoma in situ that may clinically appear like solar lentigo or other benign lesions but requires careful dermoscopic examination to identify. If the cancerous cells have broken through the basement membrane and grow deeper, it becomes a lentigo maligna melanoma. They typically arise in areas of sun damage such as the face and neck. Dermoscopically, there may be

Fig. 15.12 Melanoma in situ. Irregular pigment network, asymmetrical, disrupted borders

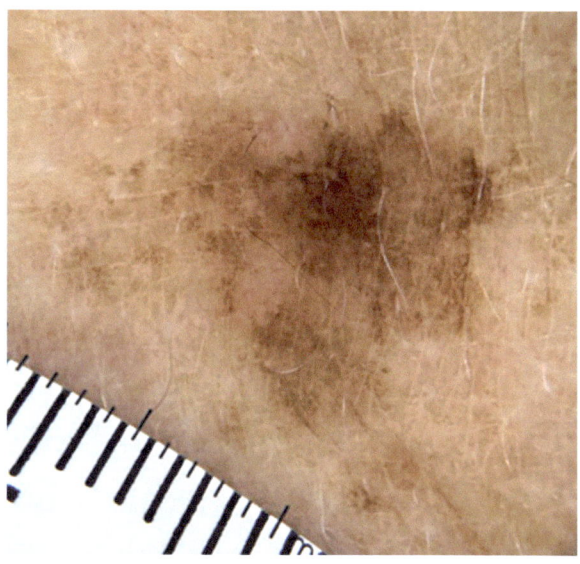

asymmetrical follicular pigmentation where pigment is only on one side of a follicular opening. If the asymmetrical pigmentation merges to surround the follicular openings, they form rhomboid structures if on the face or polygons if elsewhere on the body [29, 76]. Stolz et al. describe diagnostic criteria for facial lentigo maligna and lentigo maligna melanoma: annular-granular pattern, slate-gray dots and globules, asymmetric pigmented follicular openings, absence of criteria for flat seborrheic keratoses, and asymmetric changes over time [77]. Using these criteria in 125 cases of proven lentigo maligna melanoma, 87% were found to have at least one criterion, 69% had rhomboid structures, and 51% were found to have pigmented follicular openings [78].

Superficial Spreading and Nodular Melanoma

Superficial spreading melanoma is the most common subtype of melanoma and predominantly undergoes radial growth within the epidermis before eventually growing deeper. Dermoscopically, superficial spreading melanoma may present with high-risk features such as asymmetry, three or more colors, irregular dots/globules, irregular streaks, asymmetrical follicular pigmentation, and blue-white veil [79] (Figs. 15.13, 15.14 and 15.15).

Nodular melanoma, in contrast, tends to grow deeper into the skin relatively early with little radial growth. Because of this, nodular melanomas are responsible for a disproportionately high fraction of melanoma mortality [80]. The growth pattern also means that many dermoscopic features of melanocytic lesions such as a pigment network, dots/globules, and streaks are less likely to be seen. Instead, features of deeper skin lesions are seen: the blue color of melanin in the dermis, white

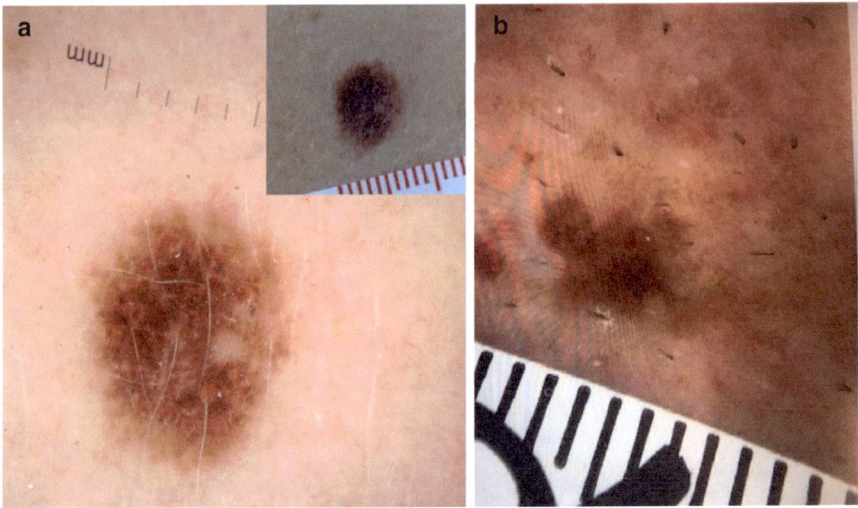

Fig. 15.13 Stage 1A superficial spreading melanoma. (**a**) shows an irregular pigment network with asymmetry. (**b**) shows a lesion with multiple patterns and irregular borders

Fig. 15.14 Stage 1A Superficial spreading melanoma. Irregular structure, hypopigmented, polymorphous vessels in pink structureless background

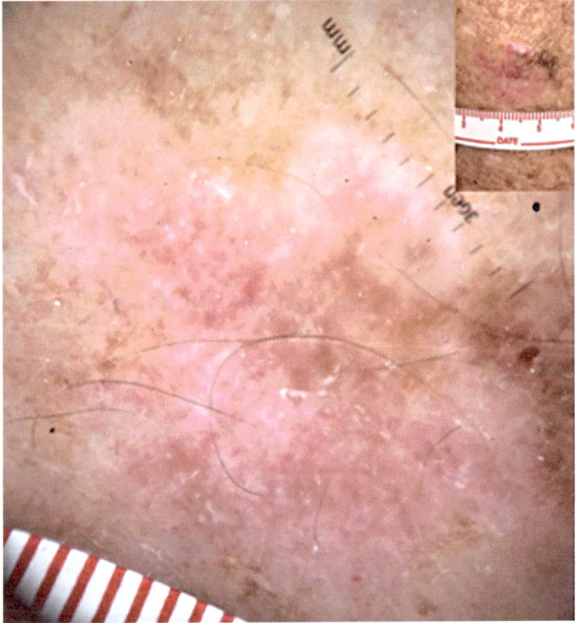

Fig. 15.15 Stage IIA superficial spreading melanoma. Irregular pigment network and structure, asymmetry, colors suggesting deeper tumor (blue/gray)

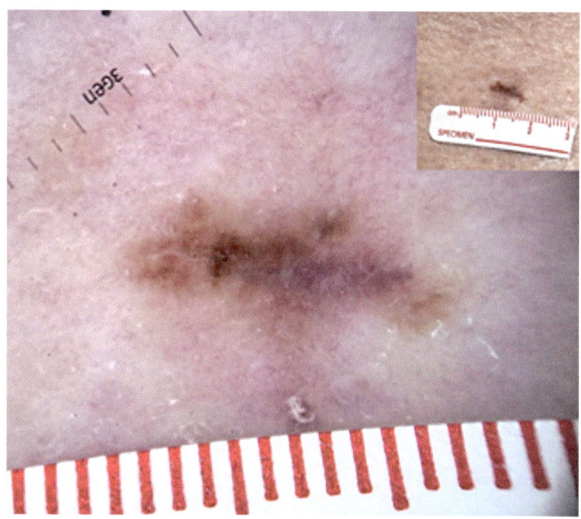

signifying regression, pink representing inflammation, and polymorphous vessels. The overlap of pigment from the depth of the lesion may lead to irregular dark brown or black blotches. It is important to note that nodular melanoma is also most likely of the various types of melanoma to present as amelanotic or hypomelanotic [81].

Hypomelanotic and Amelanotic Melanoma

Melanoma may present with little clinically visible pigment (hypomelanotic melanoma) or no clinically visible pigment (amelanotic melanoma) (Fig. 15.16). The pathogenesis may be due to downregulation of enzymes of melanin formation, such as tyrosinase [82]. This deficit in melanin means that these melanomas might not have the typical features of melanocytic lesions. Instead, it may present with mostly different shades of pink or red. Any subtype of melanoma can be hypomelanotic or amelanotic. If there are regions with melanin pigment, it is important to look for high-risk features such as asymmetry of color and structure, blue-white veil, blue-gray dots/globules, regression, and multiple components throughout the lesion [83]. Scar-like depigmentation also appears to be a positive predictor [84, 85]. In areas lacking pigmentation, the presence of irregular dot vessels (mostly in flat lesions), linear vessels (mostly in raised lesions), polymorphous vessels, or centrally located vessels suggest that the lesion is a melanoma [84, 86].

Fig. 15.16 Amelanotic melanoma. Pink structureless area, light pigmentation at periphery, dot and polymorphous vessels, ulceration

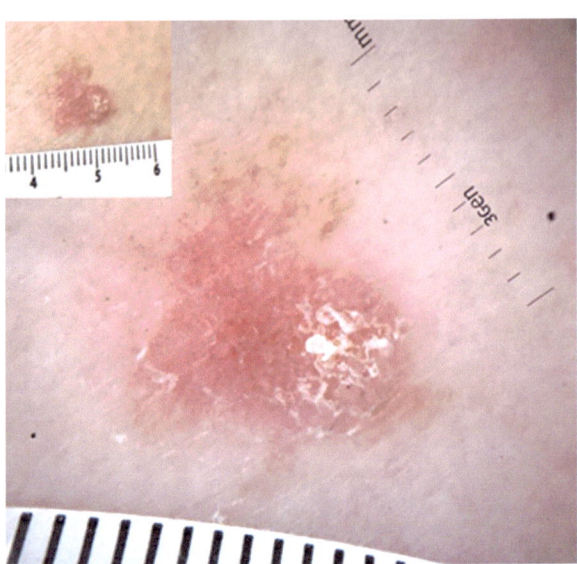

Cutaneous Metastatic Melanoma

Once a melanoma has developed to the point of metastasis, it is likely to have developed several mutations that cause it to look atypical. A cutaneous metastatic melanoma may or may not have pigment and can have varying sizes, shapes, colors, or other criteria (Fig. 15.17). Some of the most significant elements are homogeneous saccular and polymorphic atypical vascular patterns, with light brown pigmented halos and peripheral gray spots [87–89]. In amelanotic cutaneous melanoma metastases, the most predominant dermoscopic features include serpentine (45%), glomerular (30%), irregular hairpin (23%), and corkscrew vessels (19%) [90].

Acral Melanoma

Melanocytic pigment in lesions of the palms or soles follows the parallel lines of these surfaces. Benign nevi on the acral surfaces have pigment predominantly in the narrow furrows/fissures and can have bridging perpendicular lines forming a lattice-like or ladder-like pattern. Acral melanomas, on the other hand, have most of the pigment in the broad ridges with much less pigment in the furrows, producing a parallel ridge pattern [91] (Fig. 15.18). Sometimes the pigment fills both the furrows and the ridges. In these cases, it is helpful to look more peripherally where the pigment tends to fade and determine if the pigment there is mostly in the furrows or the ridges. Other features that suggest malignancy include a multicomponent pigmentation pattern, diffuse pigmentation of varying shades of brown, and milky red areas [92]. Lallas et al. propose a scoring system named BRAAFF for six variables where a total score of ≥1 is needed to diagnose acral melanoma: [B] irregular blotch

Melanoma

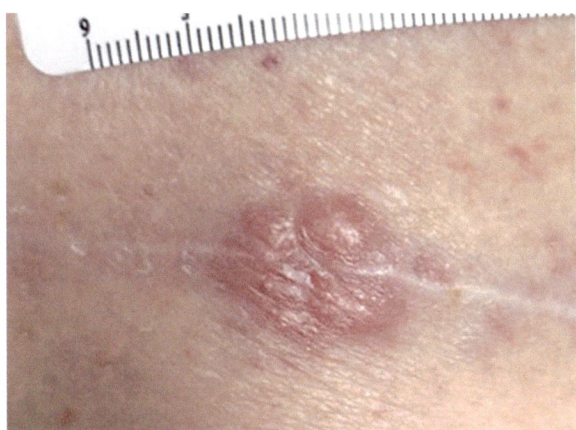

Fig. 15.17 Cutaneous metastatic melanoma

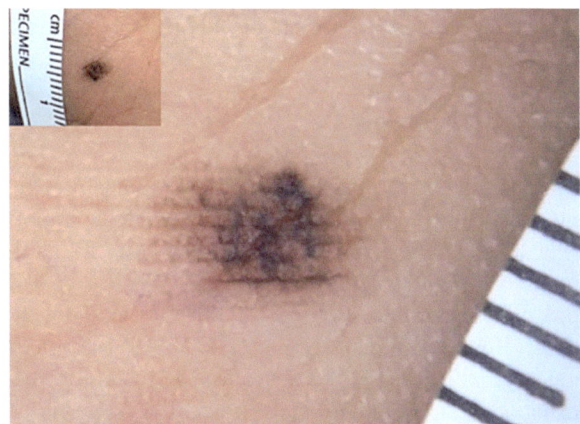

Fig. 15.18 Acral nevus. Lines parallel with pigment in furrows and pigment crosses at the ridges centrally

+1, [R] parallel ridge pattern +3, [A] asymmetry of structures +1, [A] asymmetry of colors +1, [F] parallel furrow pattern −1, and [F] fibrillar pattern −1 [93].

Subungual Melanoma

Longitudinal bands of pigment along the nail, or melanonychia, can be associated with melanocytic lesions. Benign lesions tend to produce uniform, brown-colored parallel longitudinal lines. Malignant lesions tend to have loss of parallelism, involve the first digit, involve more than two-thirds of the nail plate, and have multiple shades of brown, black, or gray [94]. They may seem irregular and if it changes over time, a histopathologic evaluation is strongly suggested. The Hutchinson sign is the extension of pigment to involve the skin either proximal or lateral to the nail plate and has good specificity for subungual melanoma [95]. Fungal melanonychia

Fig. 15.19 Mucosal nevus. Uniform pigmentation with pseudopigment (subcorneal blood, keratin, hemosiderin, or other causes) producing a darkened area. No regular pigment network is seen

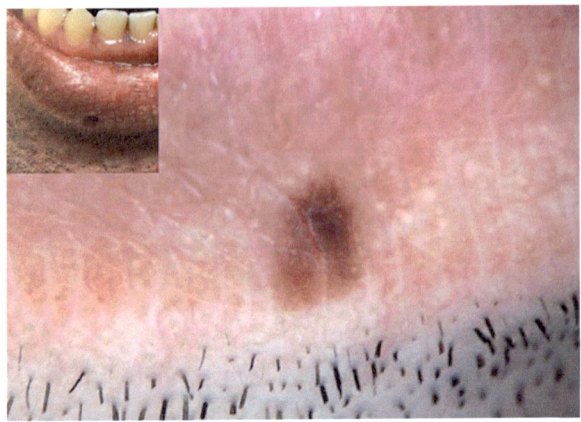

is in the differential diagnosis because melanin can also be produced, but the pattern here tends to be broader more distally because that is the origin of infection [96].

Mucosal Melanoma

Mucosal melanomas most often present clinically as a solitary brown to black macule that closely resembles the much more common finding of melanosis [97] (Fig. 15.19). One series of dermoscopic cases found that 6/8 (75%) mucosal melanomas had a multicomponent pattern, while benign lesions were found to have various patterns: dotted-globular (8/32, 25%), homogeneous (6/32, 19%), ring-like (3/32, 9%), and fingerprint-like (1/32, 3%) [98]. A review of dermoscopy use in mucosal melanoma found the following features to be useful in detecting mucosal melanoma: structureless areas, blue-white veil, multicomponent pattern, multiple colors, and irregular vessels [97].

Conclusion

Cutaneous lesions present with a wide range of possibilities and close examination with dermoscopy for the features discussed in this chapter will help clinicians classify lesions that may otherwise be ambiguous. Dermoscopy becomes a powerful tool in guiding the decision of which lesions might require further evaluation and which just need reassurance.

References

1. Richard MA, Grob JJ, Avril MF, Delaunay M, Thirion X, Wolkenstein P, et al. Melanoma and tumor thickness: challenges of early diagnosis. Arch Dermatol. 1999;135(3):269–74.

References

2. Nachbar F, Stolz W, Merkle T, Cognetta AB, Vogt T, Landthaler M, et al. The ABCD rule of dermatoscopy. High prospective value in the diagnosis of doubtful melanocytic skin lesions. J Am Acad Dermatol. 1994;30(4):551–9.
3. Argenziano G, Soyer HP. Dermoscopy of pigmented skin lesions—a valuable tool for early diagnosis of melanoma. Lancet Oncol. 2001;2(7):443–9.
4. Soyer HP, Argenziano G, Talamini R, Chimenti S. Is dermoscopy useful for the diagnosis of melanoma? Arch Dermatol. 2001;137(10):1361–3.
5. Bafounta ML, Beauchet A, Aegerter P, Saiag P. Is dermoscopy (epiluminescence microscopy) useful for the diagnosis of melanoma? Results of a meta-analysis using techniques adapted to the evaluation of diagnostic tests. Arch Dermatol. 2001;137(10):1343–50.
6. Kittler H, Pehamberger H, Wolff K, Binder M. Diagnostic accuracy of dermoscopy. Lancet Oncol. 2002;3(3):159–65.
7. Banky JP, Kelly JW, English DR, Yeatman JM, Dowling JP. Incidence of new and changed nevi and melanomas detected using baseline images and dermoscopy in patients at high risk for melanoma. Arch Dermatol. 2005;141(8):998–1006.
8. Argenziano G, Soyer HP, Chimenti S, Talamini R, Corona R, Sera F, et al. Dermoscopy of pigmented skin lesions: results of a consensus meeting via the internet. J Am Acad Dermatol. 2003;48(5):679–93.
9. Woltsche N, Schmid-Zalaudek K, Deinlein T, Rammel K, Hofmann-Wellenhof R, Zalaudek I. Abundance of the benign melanocytic universe: dermoscopic–histopathological correlation in nevi. J Dermatol. 2017;44(5):499–506.
10. Massi D, De Giorgi V, Soyer HP. Histopathologic correlates of dermoscopic criteria. Dermatol Clin. 2001;19(2):259–68. vii
11. Li Q-X, Swanson DL, Tu P, Yang S-X, Li H. Clinical and dermoscopic features of surgically treated melanocytic nevi: a retrospective study of 1046 cases. Chin Med J. 2019;132(17):2027–32.
12. de Carvalho N, Farnetani F, Ciardo S, Ruini C, Witkowski AM, Longo C, et al. Reflectance confocal microscopy correlates of dermoscopic patterns of facial lesions help to discriminate lentigo maligna from pigmented nonmelanocytic macules. Br J Dermatol. 2015;173(1):128–33.
13. Saida T, Koga H, Uhara H. Key points in dermoscopic differentiation between early acral melanoma and acral nevus. J Dermatol. 2011;38(1):25–34.
14. Kenet RO, Kang S, Kenet BJ, Fitzpatrick TB, Sober AJ, Barnhill RL. Clinical diagnosis of pigmented lesions using digital epiluminescence microscopy. Grading protocol and atlas. Arch Dermatol. 1993;129(2):157–74.
15. Soyer HP, Kenet RO, Wolf IH, Kenet BJ, Cerroni L. Clinicopathological correlation of pigmented skin lesions using dermoscopy. Eur J Dermatol. 2000;10(1):22–8.
16. Yélamos O, Braun RP, Liopyris K, Wolner ZJ, Kerl K, Gerami P, et al. Dermoscopy and dermatopathology correlates of cutaneous neoplasms. J Am Acad Dermatol. 2019;80(2):341–63.
17. Menzies SW, Crotty KA, McCarthy WH. The morphologic criteria of the pseudopod in surface microscopy. Arch Dermatol. 1995;131(4):436–40.
18. Podolec K, Bronikowska A, Pirowska M, Wojas-Pelc A. Dermoscopic features in different dermatopathological stages of cutaneous melanomas. Adv Dermatol Allergol Dermatol Alergol. 2020;37(5):677–84.
19. High WA, Francesco Tomasini C, Argenziano G, Zalaudek I. Basic principles of dermatology. In: Dermatology. 4th ed. Elsevier Limited; 2018. p. 1–43.
20. Celebi ME, Iyatomi H, Stoecker WV, Moss RH, Rabinovitz HS, Argenziano G, et al. Automatic detection of blue-white veil and related structures in dermoscopy images. Comput Med Imaging Graph. 2008;32(8):670–7.
21. Han A, Chien AL, Kang S. Photoaging. Dermatol Clin. 2014;32(3):291–9. vii
22. Praetorius C, Sturm RA, Steingrimsson E. Sun-induced freckling: ephelides and solar lentigines. Pigment Cell Melanoma Res. 2014;27(3):339–50.
23. Goorochurn R, Viennet C, Granger C, Fanian F, Varin-Blank N, Roy CL, et al. Biological processes in solar lentigo: insights brought by experimental models. Exp Dermatol. 2016;25(3):174–7.

24. Yamada T, Hasegawa S, Inoue Y, Date Y, Arima M, Yagami A, et al. Comprehensive analysis of melanogenesis and proliferation potential of melanocyte lineage in solar lentigines. J Dermatol Sci. 2014;73(3):251–7.
25. Bolognia JL. Reticulated black solar Lentigo ('Ink Spot' Lentigo). Arch Dermatol. 1992;128(7):934–40.
26. Argenziano G. Dermoscopy of melanocytic hyperplasias: subpatterns of lentigines (ink spot). Arch Dermatol. 2004;140(6):776.
27. Byrom L, Barksdale S, Weedon D, Muir J. Unstable solar lentigo: a defined separate entity. Australas J Dermatol. 2016;57(3):229–34.
28. Papageorgiou V, Apalla Z, Sotiriou E, Papageorgiou C, Lazaridou E, Vakirlis S, et al. The limitations of dermoscopy: false-positive and false-negative tumours. J Eur Acad Dermatol Venereol. 2018;32(6):879–88.
29. Tanaka M, Sawada M, Kobayashi K. Key points in dermoscopic differentiation between lentigo maligna and solar lentigo. J Dermatol. 2011;38(1):53–8.
30. Lin J, Han S, Cui L, Song Z, Gao M, Yang G, et al. Evaluation of dermoscopic algorithm for seborrhoeic keratosis: a prospective study in 412 patients. J Eur Acad Dermatol Venereol. 2014;28(7):957–62.
31. Minagawa A. Dermoscopy–pathology relationship in seborrheic keratosis. J Dermatol. 2017;44(5):518–24.
32. Zalaudek I, Kreusch J, Giacomel J, Ferrara G, Catricalà C, Argenziano G. How to diagnose nonpigmented skin tumors: a review of vascular structures seen with dermoscopy: part II. Nonmelanocytic skin tumors. J Am Acad Dermatol. 2010;63(3):377–86. quiz 387–8
33. Jin H, Yang M-Y, Kim J-M, Kim G-W, Kim H-S, Ko H-C, et al. Arborizing vessels on dermoscopy in various skin diseases other than basal cell carcinoma. Ann Dermatol. 2017;29(3):288–94.
34. Menzies SW, Westerhoff K, Rabinovitz H, Kopf AW, McCarthy WH, Katz B. Surface microscopy of pigmented basal cell carcinoma. Arch Dermatol. 2000;136(8):1012–6.
35. Higgins JC, Maher MH, Douglas MS. Diagnosing common benign skin tumors. Am Fam Physician. 2015;92(7):601–7.
36. Zaballos P, Ara M, Puig S, Malvehy J. Dermoscopy of sebaceous hyperplasia. Arch Dermatol. 2005;141(6):808.
37. Oztas P, Polat M, Oztas M, Alli N, Ustun H. Bonbon toffee sign: a new dermatoscopic feature for sebaceous hyperplasia. J Eur Acad Dermatol Venereol. 2008;22(10):1200–2.
38. Zaballos P, Gómez-Martín I, Martin JM, Bañuls J. Dermoscopy of adnexal tumors. Dermatol Clin. 2018;36(4):397–412.
39. Argenziano G, Zalaudek I, Corona R, Sera F, Cicale L, Petrillo G, et al. Vascular structures in skin tumors: a dermoscopy study. Arch Dermatol. 2004;140(12):1485–9.
40. Agero ALC, Taliercio S, Dusza SW, Salaro C, Chu P, Marghoob AA. Conventional and polarized dermoscopy features of dermatofibroma. Arch Dermatol. 2006;142(11):1431–7.
41. Warszawik-Hendzel O, Olszewska M, Maj M, Rakowska A, Czuwara J, Rudnicka L. Non-invasive diagnostic techniques in the diagnosis of squamous cell carcinoma. J Dermatol Case Rep. 2015;9(4):89–97.
42. Werner RN, Sammain A, Erdmann R, Hartmann V, Stockfleth E, Nast A. The natural history of actinic keratosis: a systematic review. Br J Dermatol. 2013;169(3):502–18.
43. Combalia A, Carrera C. Squamous cell carcinoma: an update on diagnosis and treatment. Dermatol Pract Concept. 2020;10(3):e2020066.
44. Papageorgiou C, Apalla Z, Variaah G, Matiaki FC, Sotiriou E, Vakirlis E, et al. Accuracy of dermoscopic criteria for the differentiation between superficial basal cell carcinoma and Bowen's disease. J Eur Acad Dermatol Venereol. 2018;32(11):1914–9.
45. Rosendahl C, Cameron A, Argenziano G, Zalaudek I, Tschandl P, Kittler H. Dermoscopy of squamous cell carcinoma and keratoacanthoma. Arch Dermatol. 2012;148(12):1386–92.
46. Tannous ZS, Mihm MC, Sober AJ, Duncan LM. Congenital melanocytic nevi: clinical and histopathologic features, risk of melanoma, and clinical management. J Am Acad Dermatol. 2005;52(2):197–203.

47. Odorici G, Longhitano S, Kaleci S, Chester J, Ciardo S, Pellacani G, et al. Morphology of congenital nevi in dermoscopy and reflectance confocal microscopy according to age: a pilot study. J Eur Acad Dermatol Venereol. 2020;34(12):e787–9.
48. Cengiz FP, Emiroglu N, Ozkaya DB, Su O, Onsun N. Dermoscopic features of small, medium, and large-sized congenital melanocytic nevi. Ann Dermatol. 2017;29(1):26–32.
49. Errichetti E, Patriarca MM, Stinco G. Dermoscopy of congenital melanocytic nevi: a ten-year follow-up study and comparative analysis with acquired melanocytic nevi arising in prepubertal age. Eur J Dermatol. 2017;27(5):505–10.
50. Lodha R, McDonald WS, Elgart GW, Thaller S. Dermoscopy for congenital melanocytic nevi. J Craniofac Surg. 2003;14(5):661–5.
51. Bittencourt FV, Marghoob AA, Kopf AW, Koenig KL, Bart RS. Large congenital melanocytic nevi and the risk for development of malignant melanoma and neurocutaneous melanocytosis. Pediatrics. 2000;106(4):736–41.
52. Hori Y, Nakayama J, Okamoto M, Nagae S, Taniguchi S, Takayama O, et al. Giant congenital nevus and malignant melanoma. J Invest Dermatol. 1989;92(5 Suppl):310S–4S.
53. Asdigian NL, Barón AE, Morelli JG, Mokrohisky ST, Aalborg J, Dellavalle RP, et al. Trajectories of nevus development from age 3 to 16 years in the Colorado Kids Sun Care Program Cohort. JAMA Dermatol. 2018;154(11):1272–80.
54. Kaushik A, Natsis N, Gordon SC, Seiverling EV. A practical review of dermoscopy for pediatric dermatology part I: melanocytic growths. Pediatr Dermatol. 2020;37(5):789–97.
55. Haliasos EC, Kerner M, Jaimes N, Zalaudek I, Malvehy J, Hofmann-Wellenhof R, et al. Dermoscopy for the pediatric dermatologist part III: dermoscopy of melanocytic lesions. Pediatr Dermatol. 2013;30(3):281–93.
56. Yus ES, del Cerro M, Simón RS, Herrera M, Rueda M. Unna's and Miescher's nevi: two different types of intradermal nevus: hypothesis concerning their histogenesis. Am J Dermatopathol. 2007;29(2):141–51.
57. Ackerman AB, Magana-Garcia M. Naming acquired melanocytic nevi. Unna's, Miescher's, Spitz's Clark's. Am J Dermatopathol. 1990;12(2):193–209.
58. Niederkorn A, Ahlgrimm-Siess V, Fink-Puches R, Wolf IH, Richtig E, Lackner HK, et al. Frequency, clinical and dermoscopic features of benign papillomatous melanocytic naevi (Unna type). Br J Dermatol. 2009;161(3):510–4.
59. Blum A, Hofmann-Wellenhof R, Marghoob AA, Argenziano G, Cabo H, Carrera C, et al. Recurrent melanocytic nevi and melanomas in dermoscopy: results of a multicenter study of the International Dermoscopy Society. JAMA Dermatol. 2014;150(2):138–45.
60. Botella-Estrada R, Nagore E, Sopena J, Cremades A, Alfaro A, Sanmartín O, et al. Clinical, dermoscopy and histological correlation study of melanotic pigmentations in excision scars of melanocytic tumours. Br J Dermatol. 2006;154(3):478–84.
61. Goodson AG, Florell SR, Boucher KM, Grossman D. Low rates of clinical recurrence after biopsy of benign to moderately dysplastic melanocytic nevi. J Am Acad Dermatol. 2010;62(4):591–6.
62. Tallon B, Snow J. Low clinically significant rate of recurrence in benign nevi. Am J Dermatopathol. 2012;34(7):706–9.
63. Hocker TL, Alikhan A, Comfere NI, Peters MS. Favorable long-term outcomes in patients with histologically dysplastic nevi that approach a specimen border. J Am Acad Dermatol. 2013;68(4):545–51.
64. Rosendahl CO, Grant-Kels JM, Que SKT. Dysplastic nevus: fact and fiction. J Am Acad Dermatol. 2015;73(3):507–12.
65. Kittler H, Tschandl P. Dysplastic nevus: why this term should be abandoned in dermatoscopy. Dermatol Clin. 2013;31(4):579–88. viii
66. Ardakani NM. Dysplastic/Clark naevus in the era of molecular pathology. Australas J Dermatol. 2019;60(3):186–91.
67. Kmetz EC, Sanders H, Fisher G, Lang PG, Maize JC. The role of observation in the management of atypical nevi. South Med J. 2009;102(1):45–8.

68. Kim CC, Berry EG, Marchetti MA, Swetter SM, Lim G, Grossman D, et al. Risk of subsequent cutaneous melanoma in moderately dysplastic nevi Excisionally biopsied but with positive histologic margins. JAMA Dermatol. 2018;154(12):1401–8.
69. Hofmann-Wellenhof R, Marghoob AA, Zalaudek I. Large acquired nevus or dysplastic nevus: what's in the name of a nevus? JAMA Dermatol. 2016;152(6):623–4.
70. de Brito MHTS, Dionísio CSNDM, Fernandes CMBM, Ferreira JCM, Rosa MJMDPMDC, Garcia MMAPDS. Synchronous melanomas arising within nevus spilus. An Bras Dermatol. 2017;92(1):107–9.
71. Menon K, Dusza SW, Marghoob AA, Halpern AC, Nehal KS. Classification and prevalence of pigmented lesions in patients with total-body photographs at high risk of developing melanoma. J Cutan Med Surg. 2006;10(2):85–91.
72. Kaminska-Winciorek G. Dermoscopy of nevus spilus. Dermatologic Surg. 2013;39(10):1550–4.
73. Lallas A, Apalla Z, Ioannides D, Lazaridou E, Kyrgidis A, Broganelli P, et al. Update on dermoscopy of spitz/reed naevi and management guidelines by the International Dermoscopy Society. Br J Dermatol. 2017;177(3):645–55.
74. Zalaudek I, Grinschgl S, Argenziano G, Marghoob AA, Blum A, Richtig E, et al. Age-related prevalence of dermoscopy patterns in acquired melanocytic naevi. Br J Dermatol. 2006;154(2):299–304.
75. Tlougan BE, Orlow SJ, Schaffer JV. Spitz nevi: beliefs, behaviors, and experiences of pediatric dermatologists. JAMA Dermatol. 2013;149(3):283–91.
76. Jaimes N, Marghoob AA, Rabinovitz H, Braun RP, Cameron A, Rosendahl C, et al. Clinical and dermoscopic characteristics of melanomas on nonfacial chronically sun-damaged skin. J Am Acad Dermatol. 2015;72(6):1027–35.
77. Stolz W, Schiffner R, Burgdorf WHC. Dermatoscopy for facial pigmented skin lesions. Clin Dermatol. 2002;20(3):276–8.
78. Pralong P, Bathelier E, Dalle S, Poulalhon N, Debarbieux S, Thomas L. Dermoscopy of lentigo maligna melanoma: report of 125 cases. Br J Dermatol. 2012;167(2):280–7.
79. Trindade FM, Bittencourt FV, de Freitas MLP. Dermoscopic evaluation of superficial spreading melanoma. An Bras Dermatol. 2021; [cited 2021 Feb 7]; [Internet] Available from: https://www.sciencedirect.com/science/article/pii/S0365059621000106
80. Shaikh WR, Xiong M, Weinstock MA. The contribution of nodular subtype to melanoma mortality in the United States, 1978 to 2007. Arch Dermatol. 2012;148(1):30–6.
81. Menzies SW, Moloney FJ, Byth K, Avramidis M, Argenziano G, Zalaudek I, et al. Dermoscopic evaluation of nodular melanoma. JAMA Dermatol. 2013;149(6):699–709.
82. Gong H-Z, Zheng H-Y, Li J. Amelanotic melanoma. Melanoma Res. 2019;29(3):221–30.
83. Cabrera R, Recule F. Unusual clinical presentations of malignant melanoma: a review of clinical and histologic features with special emphasis on dermatoscopic findings. Am J Clin Dermatol. 2018;19(Suppl 1):15–23.
84. Menzies SW, Kreusch J, Byth K, Pizzichetta MA, Marghoob A, Braun R, et al. Dermoscopic evaluation of amelanotic and hypomelanotic melanoma. Arch Dermatol. 2008;144(9):1120–7.
85. Bories N, Dalle S, Debarbieux S, Balme B, Ronger-Savlé S, Thomas L. Dermoscopy of fully regressive cutaneous melanoma. Br J Dermatol. 2008;158(6):1224–9.
86. Stojkovic-Filipovic J, Kittler H. Dermatoscopy of amelanotic and hypomelanotic melanoma. J Dtsch Dermatol Ges. 2014;12(6):467–72.
87. Rubegni P, Lamberti A, Mandato F, Perotti R, Fimiani M. Dermoscopic patterns of cutaneous melanoma metastases. Int J Dermatol. 2014;53(4):404–12.
88. Avilés-Izquierdo JA, Ciudad-Blanco C, Sánchez-Herrero A, Mateos-Mayo A, Nieto-Benito LM, Rodríguez-Lomba E. Dermoscopy of cutaneous melanoma metastases: a color-based pattern classification. J Dermatol. 2019;46(7):564–9.
89. Bono R, Giampetruzzi AR, Concolino F, Puddu P, Scoppola A, Sera F, et al. Dermoscopic patterns of cutaneous melanoma metastases. Melanoma Res. 2004;14(5):367–73.
90. Jaimes N, Halpern JA, Puig S, Malvehy J, Myskowski PL, Braun RP, et al. Dermoscopy: an aid to the detection of amelanotic cutaneous melanoma metastases. Dermatol Surg. 2012;38(9):1437–44.

91. Saida T, Miyazaki A, Oguchi S, Ishihara Y, Yamazaki Y, Murase S, et al. Significance of dermoscopic patterns in detecting malignant melanoma on acral volar skin: results of a multicenter study in Japan. Arch Dermatol. 2004;140(10):1233–8.
92. Braun RP, Thomas L, Dusza SW, Gaide O, Menzies S, Dalle S, et al. Dermoscopy of acral melanoma: a multicenter study on behalf of the international dermoscopy society. Dermatol Basel Switz. 2013;227(4):373–80.
93. Lallas A, Kyrgidis A, Koga H, Moscarella E, Tschandl P, Apalla Z, et al. The BRAAFF checklist: a new dermoscopic algorithm for diagnosing acral melanoma. Br J Dermatol. 2015;173(4):1041–9.
94. Benati E, Ribero S, Longo C, Piana S, Puig S, Carrera C, et al. Clinical and dermoscopic clues to differentiate pigmented nail bands: an International Dermoscopy Society study. J Eur Acad Dermatol Venereol. 2017;31(4):732–6.
95. Sohng C, Han MH, Park D, Park KD, Jang YH, Lee WJ, et al. Clinical features of subungual melanoma according to the extent of Hutchinson's nail sign: a retrospective single-centre study. J Eur Acad Dermatol Venereol. 2021;35(2):380–6.
96. Finch J, Arenas R, Baran R. Fungal melanonychia. J Am Acad Dermatol. 2012;66(5):830–41.
97. De Pascalis A, Perrot JL, Tognetti L, Rubegni P, Cinotti E. Review of dermoscopy and reflectance confocal microscopy features of the mucosal melanoma. Diagnostics. 2021;11(1):91.
98. Lin J, Koga H, Takata M, Saida T. Dermoscopy of pigmented lesions on mucocutaneous junction and mucous membrane. Br J Dermatol. 2009;161(6):1255–61.

Risk Factors for Melanoma Development 16

Risk Factors

Melanoma risk factors include both non-modifiable and modifiable factors. Table 16.1 summarizes the relative risk factors for developing melanoma [1–5]:

Tanning-bed use has also been observed to confer a slight risk to the development of melanoma. Studies indicate an OR of 1.3, which can be explained by increased exposure to UV light; however, this effect appears statistically nonsignificant after adjusting for additional factors [2].

The risk for a patient in multiple categories will be higher than that of an individual in one or none of the above categories. For modifiable risk factors like sunburns and UV exposure, activity modification and sunscreen application can be used to reduce the risk of melanoma.

Age also plays an important role in melanoma risk. For patients younger than 40 years of age, only <1 out of 200,000 moles will transform to melanoma per year. For men older than 60 years, this transformation rate increases to about 1 in 33,000 moles per year [6].

Genetic risk factors have been identified for melanoma. For those with familial history, mutations in the CDKN2A/p16 gene located on chromosome 9p21 have been implicated in melanoma development. Literature describes that pathogenic variants of CDKN2A account for 35–40% of familial melanomas with one British study finding 60–71% penetrance and 100% penetrance for families with 4–6 cases and 7–10 cases, respectively [7]. In general, carriers of pathogenic CDK2NA were younger at diagnosis and at an increased risk of developing additional melanomas [7]. Patients with xeroderma pigmentosum (XP) have defective DNA repair and experience a 1000-fold increase in melanoma risk and decreased age of onset [7].

Table 16.1 Melanoma risk factors

Risk factor	Odds ratio (95% CI)
Hair color [5]	
Black/brown	1
Blonde	1.41 (1.19–1.67)
Red	1.76 (1.41–2.16)
Nevi [3]	
0–10	1
11–50	1.7 (1.3–2.4)
51–100	3.7 (2.1–6.5)
100+	7.6 (3.5–16.2)
Atypical nevi [3]	
None	1
1–4	1.6 (1.1–2.3)
5+	6.1 (2.3–16.1)
Large nevi (≥5 mm) [5]	
None	1
1–2	2.26 (1.29–3.68)
3+	4.10 (2.19–7.08)
Sunburns [5]	
Yes	1.28 (1.05–1.27)
Familial history [5]	
Yes	1.74 (1.21–2.46)

Data from Garbe C et al. [3] and Davies JR et al. [5]

Role of Dermoscopy

Dermoscopy has an important role in facilitating diagnosis and improving the early detection of melanoma by revealing underlying structures not visible to the naked eye. Studies have demonstrated a 10–27% increase in accuracy versus diagnosis without dermoscopic tools in an experience dependent fashion [8, 9]. With proper training, dermoscopy yields high sensitivity of 68–96% and high specificity of 58–100% across multiple studies [9].

Role of Total Body Photography (TBP)

TBP helps clinicians identify new and changing lesions by enabling photographic comparisons of patient lesions across multiple time points. It has also been shown to increase the efficiency of biopsy in a study of 309 patients with risk factors for melanoma. Out of 573 suspicious changes identified, 71 were excised and 1/3 of those were revealed melanoma. This is compared to lower rates of 1/12 or 1/30 for biopsies ordered by clinicians assessing suspicious lesions without the aid of photography and dermoscopy [10].

Occupational Risk Factors

Existing literature on occupational risk factors for melanoma primarily centers on occupational sun exposure. Despite this focus, there is still disagreement regarding whether occupational sun exposure confers an increased [11], decreased [12, 13], or unchanged risk [14, 15] in melanoma incidence. Additionally, studies found other variables with far larger predictive value than sun exposure for the general working population. Of those, educational attainment is particularly significant exhibiting a positive correlation with melanoma incidence [16].

Though a general consensus does not currently exist for sun exposure, there are studies that successfully explore occupation-specific risk factors. For agricultural workers, a population that experiences increased melanoma incidence [17], pesticide exposure is one of these occupation-specific risks. Dennis et al. explore pesticide exposure in both commercial and non-commercial users and observe the strongest associations with specific fungicides (maneb/mancozeb) and insecticides (parathion), both which confer a 2.4 times risk increase [18].

Airline pilots and cabin crew are another population with increased risk for melanoma [19, 20]. In a meta-analysis of 19 studies, elevated incidence ratios of 2.21 and 2.22 were observed for flight staff and pilots, respectively (compared to the general population) [19]. It is hypothesized that these differences are driven by occupational exposure to UV radiation, which is capable of causing DNA damage and shown to induce melanoma [21–23]. Pilots and cabin crew are exposed to higher levels of UV radiation than the general population due to the effects of altitude [24], receiving as much UV-A radiation as a 20-min tanning-bed session would provide for every hour of flight at 30,000 feet [20].

Though studies do not agree about the role of occupational sun exposure in melanoma development, patients should still be encouraged to follow general advice regarding sensible sun exposure and sun protection while working. Further studies are needed to further investigate the effects of various occupational exposures and enable occupation-specific recommendations.

References

1. D'Arcy C, Holman J, Armstrong BK. Pigmentary traits, ethnic origin, benign nevi, and family history as risk factors for cutaneous malignant melanoma. J Natl Cancer Inst. 1984;72(2):257–66.
2. Evans RD, Kopf AW, Lew RA, Rigel DS, Bart RS, Friedman RJ, et al. Risk factors for the development of malignant melanoma-I: review of case-control studies. J Dermatol Surg Oncol. 1988;14(4):393–408.
3. Garbe C, Krüger S, Orfanos CE, Büttner P, Weiß J, Soyer HP, et al. Risk factors for developing cutaneous melanoma and criteria for identifying persons at risk: multicenter case-control study of the central malignant melanoma registry of the German Dermatological Society. J Invest Dermatol. 1994;102(5):695–9.
4. Chaudru V, Chompret A, Bressac-de Paillerets B, Spatz A, Avril M-F, Demenais F. Influence of genes, nevi, and sun sensitivity on melanoma risk in a family sample unselected by family history and in melanoma-prone families. JNCI J Natl Cancer Inst. 2004;96(10):785–95.

5. Davies JR, Chang Y, Bishop DT, Armstrong BK, Bataille V, Bergman W, et al. Development and validation of a melanoma risk score based on pooled data from 16 case–control studies. Cancer Epidemiol Biomarkers Prev. 2015; [Internet]. [cited 2019 Sep 29]; Available from: https://cebp.aacrjournals.org/content/early/2015/04/15/1055-9965.EPI-14-1062
6. Tsao H. The transformation rate of moles (melanocytic nevi) into cutaneous melanoma. Arch Dermatol. 2003;139(3):282.
7. Genetics of Skin Cancer (PDQ®)–Health Professional Version [Internet]. National Cancer Institute. 2009 [cited 2019 Sep 29]. Available from: https://www.cancer.gov/types/skin/hp/skin-genetics-pdq
8. Rubegni P, Burroni M, Andreassi A, Fimiani M. The role of dermoscopy and digital dermoscopy analysis in the diagnosis of pigmented skin lesions. Arch Dermatol. 2005;141(11). [Internet]. https://doi.org/10.1001/archderm.141.11.1444.
9. Kittler H, Pehamberger H, Wolff K, Binder M. Diagnostic accuracy of dermoscopy. Lancet Oncol. 2002;3(3):159–65.
10. Rice ZP, Weiss FJ, DeLong LK, Curiel-Lewandrowski C, Chen SC. Utilization and rationale for the implementation of total body (digital) photography as an adjunct screening measure for melanoma. Melanoma Res. 2010;1
11. Chang Y, Barrett JH, Bishop DT, Armstrong BK, Bataille V, Bergman W, et al. Sun exposure and melanoma risk at different latitudes: a pooled analysis of 5700 cases and 7216 controls. Int J Epidemiol. 2009;38(3):814–30.
12. Gandini S, Sera F, Cattaruzza MS, Pasquini P, Picconi O, Boyle P, et al. Meta-analysis of risk factors for cutaneous melanoma: II. Sun exposure. Eur J Cancer. 2005;41(1):45–60.
13. Caini S, Gandini S, Sera F, Raimondi S, Fargnoli MC, Boniol M, et al. Meta-analysis of risk factors for cutaneous melanoma according to anatomical site and clinico-pathological variant. Eur J Cancer. 2009;45(17):3054–63.
14. Kricker A, Armstrong BK, Goumas C, Litchfield M, Begg CB, Hummer AJ, et al. Ambient UV, personal sun exposure and risk of multiple primary melanomas. Cancer Causes Control. 2007;18(3):295–304.
15. Vuong K, McGeechan K, Armstrong BK, AMFS Investigators, GEM Investigators, Cust AE. Occupational sun exposure and risk of melanoma according to anatomical site. Int J Cancer. 2014;134(11):2735–41.
16. Goodman KJ, Bible ML, London S, Mack TM. Proportional melanoma incidence and occupation among White males in Los Angeles County (California, United States). Cancer Causes Control. 1995;6(5):451–9.
17. Spiewak R. Pesticides as a cause of occupational skin diseases in farmers. Ann Agric Environ Med. 2001;8(1):1–5.
18. Dennis LK, Lynch CF, Sandler DP, Alavanja MCR. Pesticide use and cutaneous melanoma in pesticide applicators in the agricultural heath study. Environ Health Perspect. 2010;118(6):812–7.
19. Sanlorenzo M, Wehner MR, Linos E, Kornak J, Kainz W, Posch C, et al. The risk of melanoma in airline pilots and cabin crew: a meta-analysis. JAMA Dermatol. 2015;151(1):51–8.
20. Sanlorenzo M, Vujic I, Posch C, Cleaver JE, Quaglino P, Ortiz-Urda S. The risk of melanoma in pilots and cabin crew: UV measurements in flying airplanes. JAMA Dermatol. 2015;151(4):450–2.
21. Gilchrest BA, Eller MS, Geller AC, Yaar M. The pathogenesis of melanoma induced by ultraviolet radiation. N Engl J Med. 1999;340(17):1341–8.
22. Ananthaswamy HN, Pierceall WE. Molecular mechanisms of ultraviolet radiation carcinogenesis. Photochem Photobiol. 1990;52(6):1119–36.
23. Ley R, Applegate L, Padilla RS, Stuart T. Ultraviolet radiation—induced malignant melanoma in Monodelphis domestica. Photochem Photobiol. 1989;50(1):1–5.
24. Nakagawara V, Montgomery R, Marshall W. Optical radiation transmittance of aircraft windscreens and pilot vision. Washington (DC): Office of Aerospace Medicine (US); 2007. Report No.:DOT/FAA/AM-07/20.

Index

A
Access to care, 104
Acquired nevus, 125
Acral lentiginous melanoma, 102
Acral melanoma, 134, 135
Acral nevus, 135
Actinic keratosis, 123
Adjunctive cryotherapy, 88
Adjuvant radiation therapy, 66
Adjuvant therapy, 25, 26, 66
Adverse events, 47–49
African Americans, 100–102, 104
Amelanotic, Bleeding or Bump, Color uniformity, De novo, any Diameter (ABCD), 51
Amelanotic melanoma, 51, 133, 134
Amelanotic nevus, 125
Anorectal melanoma, 65
Anti-CTLA-4, 42, 67
Anti-PD-1, 39, 42, 67
  therapy, 40, 58
Asians, 99
Asymmetry, Border, Color, Diameter, Evolving (ABCDE), 51
Atypical Spitz tumor (AST), 52
Azathioprine, 112

B
Basal cell carcinoma, 121, 122
Benign melanocytic lesions, 125
  acquired nevus, 125
  blue nevus, 126
  combined nevus, 126
  congenital nevus, 125
  Unna and Miescher nevi, 126
Biomarkers, 42
Blue nevus, 126
BRAF inhibitors, 7, 8, 10, 11, 38, 41, 47, 48, 58, 65, 89

BRAF V600E/K mutations, 10, 67, 89
Brain metastases, 38
BRCA1-associated protein 1 (BAP1), 79
Breslow depth, 1, 29, 103
Breslow thickness, 102

C
Cancer immunoediting, 109
Cardiac adverse events, 48
Caucasian melanoma, 101
CDK4, 18
CDKN1A, 89
CDKN2A/p16 gene, 17, 18, 143
Checkmate-067, 40
Checkmate-069, 40
Checkmate 204 trial, 40
Checkmate-511 trial, 40, 48
Chemotherapy, 38, 88, 91, 92
Chromosomal alterations, 78, 79
Ciliary body involvement, 72, 73
coBRIM phase III trial, 39, 47
COLUMBUS trial, 39
Combined nevus, 126, 127
Comparative genomic hybridization (CGH), 12, 13
Complete lymph node dissection (CLND), 25
Complete response (CR), 30–32
Compound nevi, 126
Congenital melanocytic nevi (CMN), 52–54
Congenital nevus, 125
Conjunctival melanocytic intraepithelial neoplasia (C-MIN), 87, 88, 92
Conjunctival melanoma (CoM), 87–89
  differential diagnosis, 89
  genetic abnormalities, 89, 90
  incidence, 88
  management, 91–93
  prognosis, 93, 94
  staging, 90

Cryotherapy, 91, 92
CTLA-4 inhibitor, 39, 40, 48
Cutaneous metastatic melanoma, 134, 135
Cyclin-dependent kinase N2A (CDKN2A), 7, 8, 10
Cyclin D1 protein expression, 78
Cyclophosphamide, 111

D
Dermatofibroma, 122
Dermatologic toxicities, 48
Dermoscopy, 117, 136
   benign melanocytic lesions, 125
      acquired nevus, 125
      blue nevus, 126
      combined nevus, 126
      congenital nevus, 125
      Unna and Miescher nevi, 126
   features of melanocytic lesions, 119
   higher-risk melanocytic lesions
      dysplastic nevus, 128
      nevus spilus, 129
      recurrent nevus, 127
      spitz nevus, 130
   melanoma
      acral melanoma, 134, 135
      cutaneous metastatic melanoma, 134
      hypomelanotic and amelanotic melanoma, 133
      lentigo maligna and lentigo maligna melanoma, 130, 131
      melanoma in situ, 130
      mucosal melanoma, 136
      subungual melanoma, 135, 136
      superficial spreading and nodular melanoma, 131, 133
   nonmelanocytic lesions, 120
      basal cell carcinoma, 121, 122
      dermatofibroma, 122
      ink spot lentigo, 120
      sebaceous gland hyperplasia, 122
      seborrheic keratosis, 121
      solar lentigo, 120
      squamous cell carcinoma, 123
      vascular lesions, 123
   role of, 144
   stratifying risk of melanocytic lesions, 124
Diffuse pattern, 73
Disease-free survival, 23, 24
Dysplastic nevus, 128

E
Environmental exposure, 100
Epithelioid cells, 74
European Society for Medical Oncology (ESMO), 42
Extraocular extension (EOE), 73

F
Familial melanoma
   genetic mutations, 17, 18
   genetic testing and counseling, 18, 19
Fluorescence in situ hybridization (FISH), 12, 13

G
Gene expression profiling (GEP), 79
Genetic testing, 18, 19
Genitourinary melanoma, 64
Germline mutation, 17
Glucocorticoids, 111
GNA11 mutations, 78
GNAQ protein, 78
Granulocyte-macrophage colony-stimulating factor (GM-CSF), 32

H
Head and neck mucosal melanoma, 64
Higher-risk melanocytic lesions
   dysplastic nevus, 128
   nevus spilus, 129
   recurrent nevus, 127
   spitz nevus, 130
High mitotic rate, 75
Hispanics, 99–102, 104
HMB-45, 76, 77
Hormone replacement therapy, 59
Hyperthermic isolated limb perfusion (HILP), 30, 31
Hypomelanotic melanoma, 133
Hypoxia-inducible factor 1A (HIF1A), 18

I
IL-6, 111
Immune checkpoint blockade, 67
Immune checkpoint inhibitors, 48, 49, 66, 67
   therapy, 42
Immune system, 109, 111
Immunoediting, 109

Immunohistochemical markers, 76, 77
Immunomodulator drugs, 111
Immunosuppression, 109, 111
Immunotherapy, 37, 39–42, 93, 109
Inconclusive melanoma risk, 111, 112
Inflammation, 76
Inflammatory conditions, 110
Ink spot lentigo, 120
Interleukin-2 (IL-2), 110
Intralesional Bacille Calmette-Guerin (BCG), 32
Intralesional therapy, 32, 33
In-transit melanoma, 29, 30, 32
Ipilimumab, 39, 58
Isolated limb infusion (ILI), 31
Isolated limb perfusion (ILP), 30, 31

K
Keratoacanthoma, 47
Keynote 006 trial, 48
KEYNOTE-029, 40
Ki-67, 77
KIT, 65–67

L
Largest tumor diameter, 72
Lentigines, 120
Lentigo maligna melanoma, 130, 131
Liver function tests (LFTs), 71
Lymph nodes, 2
    dissection, 25
Lymphocyte-activating gene 3 (LAG-3), 41

M
Mammalian target of rapamycin (mTOR), 110
MC1R, 18
Mean diameter of ten largest nucleoli, 74
MEK inhibitor, 38, 39, 41, 47
Melan-A, 77
Melanocytic lesions
    features of, 119
    stratifying risk of, 124
Melanocytic tumors of uncertain malignant potential (MELTUMPs), 52
Melanoma, 7
    clinical application of CGH/FISH, 12
    mutation
        effects, therapy, 10, 11
        in pathogenesis, 7–9

testing, 10
Melanoma development
    in immunosuppressed patients, 109, 110
    in non-White populations, 100, 101
    risk factors, 143
        age, 143
        genetic risk factors, 143
        modifiable risk factors, 143
        occupational risk factors, 145
        dermoscopy, 144
        tanning-bed, 143
        TBP, 144
Melanoma in situ, 130, 131
Melanoma risk
    immunosuppressed patients, melanoma development in, 109, 110
    inconclusive, 111, 112
    increased, 110
    melanoma prognosis, immunosuppressant treatment, 112, 113
    no increased, 111
    progression/recurrence, 112
Melanoma-specific survival, 23, 24, 26
Melanoma staging, 1
    lymph nodes (N), 2
        clinically detected, 2
        clinically occult, 2
        in-transit metastases, 2
        matted nodes, 2
        microsatellite metastases, 2
        pathological stage, 3
        possible N values, 3
        satellite metastases, 2
    metastatic spread (M), 3
    stage 0, 4
    stage grouping, 4
    stage IA, 4
    stage IB, 4
    stage IIA, 4
    stage IIB, 4
    stage IIC, 4
    stage IIIA, 5
    stage IIIB, 5
    stage IIIC, 5
    stage IIID, 5
    stage IV, 6
    tumor characteristics (T), 1
        mitotic count (rate), 2
        possible T values, 2
        thickness (Breslow depth), 1
        ulceration, 1
Melanosis, 87

Metastasis, 1, 3
Metastatic melanoma, 38–41
Microcirculation, 75, 76
Microphthalmia-associated transcription factor (MITF), 18
Miescher nevi, 126
Minority populations, melanoma
  clinical presentation, 101–103
  incidences and rates of melanoma death, in White and Black populations, 99
  non-White populations, melanoma development in, 100, 101
  prevention, 103, 104
Mitogen activated protein kinase (MAPK), 7–10
Mitomycin C, 88, 92
Mitotic count (rate), 2
Mixed-cell melanomas, 74
Molecular pathway defects, 78
Mucosal melanocytes, 63
Mucosal melanoma, 63, 102, 136
  adjuvant therapy, 66
  anorectal, 65
  genitourinary, 64
  head and neck, 64
  management of primary disease, 66
  molecular biology, 65, 66
  systemic therapy, 67
Mucosal nevus, 136
Multiplex ligation-dependent probe amplification (MLPA), 89
Mycophenolate mofetil, 111

N
Nasal cavity melanomas, 64
Natalizumab, 110
National Health Interview Surveys, 104
Neurofibromin 1 (NF1), 8, 10, 65
Neurologic adverse events, 48
Nevus spilus, 129
Nodular melanoma, 131
Non-Hispanic Whites (NHW), 99–102, 104
Nonirradiated melanomas, 77
Nonmelanocytic lesions, 51, 120
  basal cell carcinoma, 121, 122
  dermatofibroma, 122
  ink spot lentigo, 120
  sebaceous gland hyperplasia, 122
  seborrheic keratosis, 121
  solar lentigo, 120
  squamous cell carcinoma, 123
  vascular lesions, 123

"No touch" surgical approach, 91
NRAS, 7, 8, 10, 65

O
Occupational risk factors, 145
Ophthalmic adverse events, 48
Optic nerve involvement, 74
OPTiM randomized phase III trial, 32
Oral contraceptive pills (OCP), 59
Organ transplant recipients (OTRs), 109
Oropharyngeal primary mucosal melanoma, 64
Overall response rate (ORR), 30–33, 38
Overall survival (OS), 30, 31, 38–42

P
PD-1 inhibitors, 48
Pediatric melanoma, 51
  clinical presentation, 51, 52
  management, 54
  prognosis, 53, 54
  risk factors, 53
Personalized therapy, 42
Phospho-histone H3 (PHH3), 75
Pregnancy and melanoma
  diagnosis, 57, 59
  immunosuppressive changes, 58
  impact, 57
  influence of hormones, 59
  meta-analysis, 59
  multidisciplinary counseling, 58
  postpartum period, 59
  treatment for patients, 58
Primary acquired melanosis (PAM), 87, 93
Primary CoM, 89
Primary melanomas, 29, 109
Primary treatment, 25, 26
Progression free survival (PFS), 38–41
Protection of telomeres I (POT1), 18
PTEN, 8, 10, 11
Puberty, 52–54
Public education, 104–105
Pulmonary adverse events, 48
PV-10, 32

R
Radiotherapy, 91
Rb protein, 78
Receptor tyrosine kinase, 8
Recurrent nevus, 127

Regionally advanced melanoma
  ILI, 31
  ILP, 30, 31
  intralesional therapy, 32, 33
Regulatory T cells (Tregs), 57
RELATIVITY-047 study, 41
Ring melanoma, 73, 74
Rule of 2s, 19
Rule of 3s, 19
RUNX2, 89

S
S100, 77
Satellite metastases, 29
Sebaceous gland hyperplasia, 122
Seborrheic keratosis, 121
SECOMBIT, 42
Secondary prevention, 103, 104
Sentinel lymph node biopsy (SLNB), 23–25, 52, 54, 58, 90, 92
Serous retinopathy, 47
SF3B1, 65, 66
Side effects of melanoma therapy
  immune checkpoint inhibitors, 48, 49
  targeted therapy, 47
Sinonasal tract mucosal melanomas, 64
Sociocultural values, 104
Socioeconomic status, 104
Solar lentigines, 120
Solar lentigo, 120
Spindle cells, 74
Spitz nevi, 52, 130
Spitz nevus, 130
SPRED1, 65
Squamous cell carcinoma, 47, 123
Stage 0 treatment, 23
Stage IA treatment, 23
Stage IB–II treatment
  SLN biopsy, 23, 24
  wide local excision, 23
Stage III treatment, 25, 26
Stage IV treatment
  brain metastases, 38
  combination immunotherapy, 40, 41
  combination targeted and immuno-
    therapy, 41
  immunotherapy, 39, 40
  surgery, 37
  targeted therapy, 38, 39
Standardized incidence ratio (SIR), 110
Stereotactic radiosurgery (SRS), 38
Subungual melanoma, 135, 136

Sun protection, 104
  factor, 100
  sites, 101
Superficial spreading melanoma, 131–133
Surveillance, 25
Surveillance, Epidemiology, and End Results
    (SEER) Program, 51, 101
Survival, 23–26
Swedish Cancer and Multi-Generation
    Register, 57
Swedish National and Regional Registries, 57
Systemic IL-2, 32
Systemic inflammatory response syndrome
    (SIRS), 32
Systemic therapy, 29, 67

T
Talimogene laherparepvec (T-VEC), 32
Targeted therapy, 10, 11, 37–39, 41, 42, 47, 66, 67, 93
Telomerase reverse transcriptase (TERT), 8, 9
Therapeutic lymph node dissection
    (TLND), 25
Tocilizumab, 111
Topical chemotherapy, 88, 92
Total body photography (TBP), 144
TP53, 8, 9
Transplantation, 112
Transpupillary thermotherapy, 80
Treatment for melanoma
  baseline imaging, primary treatment and
      adjuvant treatment and
      observation, 25, 26
  SLN biopsy, 23, 24
  stage 0 treatment, 23
  stage IA treatment, 23
  stage IB–II treatment, 23, 24
  stage III treatment, 25, 26
  wide local excision, 23
TRIDeNT, 42
Tumor infiltrating lymphocytes (TILs), 39
Tumor necrosis factor alpha (TNFα)
    inhibitors, 112
Tyndall effect, 119

U
Ulceration, 1, 2, 4, 5
Unna nevi, 126, 127
Ustekinumab, 111
UV exposure, 143
UV radiation, 63

Uveal melanoma (UM), 71
   class 1, 79
   class 2, 79
   clinical high-risk features
      ciliary body involvement, 72, 73
      diffuse pattern, 73
      extraocular extension, 73
      largest tumor diameter, 72
      older age, 72
      optic nerve involvement, 74
      ring melanoma, 73, 74
   early diagnosis, 71
   histological high-risk features
      cell type, 74
      high mitotic rate, 75
      inflammation, 76
      mean diameter of the ten largest nucleoli, 74
      microcirculation, 75, 76
      pigmentation, 76
   immunohistochemical markers, 76, 77
   incidence, 71
   molecular alterations, in UM metastases, 79
   molecular pathology, 77, 78
   primary UM
      chromosomal alterations, 78, 79
      molecular pathway defects, 78
      molecular techniques, 79
   prognosis, 71, 72, 76
   risk factors, 71
   scope of prognostication, 80
   treatment modalities, 80, 81

V

Vascular lesions, 123
Vemurafenib, 38

W

Whole genome sequencing study, 66
Wide local excision
   stage 0 treatment, 23
   stage IA treatment, 23
   stage IB–II treatment, 23, 24

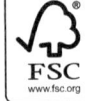

MIX
Papier aus verantwortungsvollen Quellen
Paper from responsible sources
FSC® C105338

If you have any concerns about our products,
you can contact us on
ProductSafety@springernature.com

In case Publisher is established outside the EU,
the EU authorized representative is:
Springer Nature Customer Service Center GmbH
Europaplatz 3, 69115 Heidelberg, Germany

Printed by Libri Plureos GmbH
in Hamburg, Germany